Total Revision:
Extended Paediatrics

Dr L J Michaelis BSc(Hons) MBChB MRCPCH
Specialist Paediatric Registrar
St Mary's Hospital NHS Trust
London

Dr I Maconochie MB BS FFAEM FRCPCH
Consultant in Paediatric Accident and Emergency
St Mary's Hospital NHS Trust
London

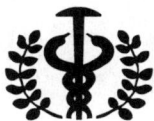

PasTest
Dedicated to your success

© 2005 PasTest Ltd
Egerton Court
Parkgate Estate
Knutsford
Cheshire, WA16 8DX

Telephone: 01565 752000

First edition 2005

ISBN: 1 904627 13 7

A catalogue record for this book is available from the British Library.

PasTest Revision Books and Intensive Courses

PasTest has been established in the field of postgraduate medical education since 1972, providing revision books and intensive study courses for doctors preparing for their professional examinations. Books and courses are available for the following specialties:

MRCP Part 1 and Part 2, MRCPCH Part 1 and Part 2, MRCOG, DRCOG, MRCGP, MRCPsych, DCH, FRCA, MRCS and PLAB.

For further details contact:

PasTest Ltd, Freepost, Knutsford, Cheshire, WA16 7BR
Tel: 01565 752000   Fax: 01565 650264
Email: enquiries@pastest.co.uk   Web site: www.pastest.co.uk

Typeset by Saxon Graphics Ltd, Derby
Printed by Alden Group Ltd, Oxfordshire

Contents

CONTENTS

Contributors

Ian Maconochie is a leading Paediatric Consultant in accident and emergency at St Mary's Hospital, Paddington, London. He lectures on many aspects of advanced paediatric life support and paediatric emergencies both in the United Kingdom and abroad. His specialist interest lies in conducting research in accident and emergency.

Louise Michaelis is a Specialist Paediatric Registrar who has an interest in immunology, allergy and infectious diseases.

Foreword

What do you get if you combine the wisdom and knowledge of a consultant paediatrician with the practical experience of a paediatric trainee who has recently overcome the daunting hurdle of postgraduate paediatric exams? – You get this pearl of a book designed to ease the trainee paediatrician over the MRCPCH part 1 (a, b) or the General Practitioner trainee wishing to demonstrate competence by passing the DCH (part a).

Ian Maconochie has provided the knowledge of the clinical scenarios on which the questions are based, and Louise Michaelis, as a trainee recently successful in the exam, and very familiar with the needs of trainees, has set out the questions in a format guaranteed to give the user an advantage over other candidates not familiar with this book.

There is no easy way to pass postgraduate exams – you need to demonstrate knowledge and competence in using that knowledge. This book helps candidates focus their learning and hone their techniques – allowing them to make the most of their hard earned knowledge and skills.

Good luck to all who use this gem of a book – and congratulations to the authors!

Dr Andrew Raffles FRCPCH DCH MBBS
Consultant Paediatrician and Clinical Director
Fellow and Examiner for the Royal College of Paediatrics and Child Health

Introduction

Total Revision: Extended Paediatrics has been written to give candidates new questions similar to those now set in the new format for the MRCPCH Part 1 and DCH examinations. The questions have been written to give students an insight into the new way of examining subject matter. The chapters have been divided into specialties. At the beginning of each chapter there is a Question Frequency List, which gives the candidate an idea of how often certain topics have been cited in the various examinations over the last five years, even when the examination was given in paediatric and adult specialties.

Since January 2004, the MRCPCH examination has consisted of two papers:

Paper 1A
The first paper focuses on conditions that any practitioner who deals with children would encounter. This includes conditions that would be seen in a hospital, community or primary care setting. This is also known as the Basic Child Health paper.

Paper 1 B
The written paper deals with more complicated problem-solving skills, with an emphasis on the scientific knowledge underpinning child health care. This is also known as the Extended Paediatric paper. This paper is equivalent to the previous MRCPCH Part 1 paper.

Candidates must pass both papers in order to proceed to sit the MRCPCH Part 2 examination.

Both Papers 1A and 1B are set for 2½ hours and comprise:
35 40–45 Multiple True/False questions   each worth 5 marks
25 17–20 Best of Five Questions   each worth 4 marks
7–9 Extended Matching Questions   each worth 9 marks (3 marks per item)

The Multiple True/False question (MTF) is the form of question with which most candidates are familiar – five separate questions under a stem with each of the five questions having a true or false answer.

The Best of Five question (BoF) has five options to match the heading statement or scenario. Of these options there is only one correct answer.

The Extended Matching Question (EMQ) has ten associated options for which three scenarios or statements are given. For each of these there is only one correct answer.

There is no negative marking, hence it is advised that all questions should be attempted.

The pass mark is calculated with regard to the predicted difficulty of each of the questions in the paper, and questions are graded into their appropriateness as being one of three categories; namely, essential, important or acceptable.

Access the RCPCH website to see examples of the examination and to keep up to date with any alteration in the examination that may occur: www.Rcpch.ac.uk

We are grateful to Annabel Thomas, Carrie Walker, Kirsten Baxter and Amy Smith for all their work and encouragement in publishing this book. We hope that you will enjoy this book and we wish you all the very best and good luck in passing the dreaded MRCPCH Examination.

Ian Maconochie
Louise Michaelis

Questions

Basic Science

Question Frequency

Adhesion molecules	0	Fluorescence in situ hybridisation	
Allergy	2	(FISH)	0
Allograft rejection	3	Free radicals	0
ALU sequence	0	G proteins	0
Angiogenesis	0	Gene cloning	0
Anti-oncogenes	0	Gene regulation	0
Antiprotein A1	0	Gene therapy	0
Antisense oligodeoxy nucleotides	0	Glycoproteins	0
Apolipoprotein E	0	Haemopoietic stem cells	0
Apoptosis	1	Heat shock proteins	0
Aquaporins	0	HMG CoA	0
Arachidonic acid	1	Hybridisation	0
Assays	0	Knockout mice	0
Associations	0	Left recurrent laryngeal nerve	0
Atrial naturetic peptide (adult)	7	Linkage	0
Atrial receptors (adult)	4	Meiosis	0
Blood flow to hands	0	Mini-satellite probing	0
Bones	0	Mitosis	0
Cell cycle	0	Monoclonal antibodies (adult)	4
Cell membrane	0	Mutator genes	0
Cellular signal transduction	0	Northern blotting	0
Cellular signalling	0	Nuclear factor	0
Codon	0	Oncogene – proto	0
Creatine kinase	1	Oncogene – ras	0
DNA	1	Oncogenes (adult)	1
DNA mutations	1	P53 gene	0
Endothelins	0	Paraproteins	0
Erythropoietin	0	Polymerase chain reaction (PCR)	
External jugular vein	0	(adult)	4

Peroxisomes	0	RNA	0
Plasma proteins	0	Southern blotting	0
Platelet activating factor	0	Tandem repeats	0
Prostacyclin (adult)	1	Transcription factors	0
Protein kinases	0	Transforming growth factor β	0
Receptor – TH cell	0	Transgenic animals	0
Receptors	3	Translation	0
Receptors – LDL receptor	0	Tumour necrosis factor (adult)	6
Receptors – T cell	2	Tumour suppressor genes (adult)	1
Restriction endonucleases	1	Tyrosine kinases	0
Retroviruses	0	Umbilical artery	0
RFLP	1	Vascular tone	1
Ribozomes	0	Viruses and cancer	0
Right recurrent laryngeal nerve	0	Western blotting	0

Multiple True/False Questions

1   **You are asked to review a treatment plan for a child who presents with left ventricular failure and hypertension. You are given the following five options for treatment. Which of these may benefit your patient?**

○ A Activating acyl-CoA : cholesterol *O*-acyltransferase (ACAT)
○ B Synthetic cachectic lymphotoxin
○ C Aldosterone
○ D Atrial natriuretic peptide (ANP)
○ E Tumour necrosis factor

2   **Atrial receptors are involved in the regulation of body fluids. They act via four mechanisms. Which of the following is *not* regulated by atrial receptors?**

○ A Stimulation of free nerve endings throughout both the left and right atria
○ B An increase in antidiuretic hormone release
○ C A decrease in renin release
○ D A decrease in aldosterone release
○ E Inhibition of sodium reabsorption in the distal nephron, causing excretion of sodium and water but not potassium

3   **Which of the following five statements refers to the technique called Southern blotting?**

○ A A demonstration of the presence or absence of specific whole *RNA* sequences in the tissues using a DNA probe
○ B A demonstration of the presence or absence of specific *DNA* fragments in a mixture of DNA
○ C The detection of a particular *protein* in a mixture
○ D The detection and presence of a fluorescence in situ *hybridisation antibody*
○ E The detection and presence of *genetic markers* using micro rays

4   **Which of the following five statements refers to the technique called Northern blotting?**

○ A A demonstration of the presence or absence of specific whole *RNA* sequences in the tissues using a *DNA* probe
○ B A demonstration of the presence or absence of specific *DNA* fragments in a mixture of DNA
○ C The detection of a particular *protein* in a mixture
○ D The detection and presence of a fluorescence in situ *hybridisation antibody*
○ E The detection and presence of *genetic markers* using micro rays

5 **Which of the following five statements refers to the technique called Western blotting?**

○ A A demonstration of the presence or absence of specific whole *RNA* sequences in the tissues using a *DNA* probe

○ B The demonstration of the presence or absence of specific *DNA* fragments in a mixture of DNA

○ C The detection of a particular *protein* in a mixture

○ D The detection and presence of a fluorescence in situ *hybridisation antibody*

○ E The detection and presence of *genetic markers* using micro rays

6 **Of the following five clinical disorders, which does *not* involve the use of monoclonal antibodies?**

○ A Monoclonal gammopathies

○ B Waldenström's macroglobulinaemia

○ C Cryoglobulinaemias

○ D Myeloma – lytic bone lesions

○ E Immunodeficiency

Best of Five Questions

7 **Which of the following medical biological processes is apoptosis *not* responsible for?**

○ A AIDS (acquired immunodeficiency syndrome)

○ B Systemic lupus erythematosus (SLE)

○ C Chicken pox

○ D *p53* mutations

○ E The overexpression of *bcl-2* in t(14:18) in haematological disease

8 **This substance is called synthetic cachectic lymphotoxin. It is a cytokine (polypeptide) that is pleiotropic; ie it has many actions. It is a pro-inflammatory cytokine and has catabolic properties in the production of bacterial toxins, inflammatory products and invasive stimuli. It acts on macrophages, eosinophils and natural killer cells, whereas the β component acts on T lymphocytes. Both bind to the same receptor and have the same actions. The α component is also a potent stimulator of prostaglandin production, and the α and β components are located on the MHCII region of chromosome 6.**

What is this substance?

- A Granulocytic colony-stimulating factor
- B Cyclic adenosine monophosphate (cAMP)
- C Tumour necrosis factor (TNF)
- D Atrial natriuretic peptide
- E Tyrosine kinase

Extended Matching Question

9 Theme: Receptors

- A Ligand-gated receptor
- B Protein tyrosine kinase activated receptor
- C G-protein-coupled receptor
- D Steroid receptor
- E T cell receptor (TCR)
- F Low-density lipoprotein (LDL) receptor
- G Vitamin D receptor
- H H2 receptor
- I FbGF3 receptor
- J Growth hormone receptor

For the ten receptors listed, state which is described in each of the three clinical scenarios below.

1 This receptor is a dimer and is part of the CD3 complex. It is an intracellular cell wall receptor like the steroid receptors. It detects antigen in association with human leukocyte antigen (HLA) molecules, and works within the nucleoplasm membrane and the mitochondria. It is activated by antigen binding, and activation of the intracellular signal transduction pathway subsequently exists. It increases interleukin-2 levels but does not interact with the CD3 complex per se. Which receptor is this?

2 This receptor is part of the superantigen family. It has a similar action and structure to the thyroid and vitamin D receptors. It is located on the intracellular cell wall. It works within the cytoplasmic environment and is known as a nuclear hormone. When the chemical reacts with the ligand, it binds with DNA and not RNA to cause an effect. This receptor is not stabilised by heat shock proteins. It is not blocked by aminoglutethimide, which inhibits the conversion of androgens to oestrogens in tissues. What is this receptor?

3 This receptor is associated with abnormalities of chromosome 19. A mutation concerning this receptor can lead to the clinical syndrome of familial hypercholesterolaemia. It is not restricted to the cell surface

and continuously recycles from the cell surface to the endosomes, internalising its molecules for catabolism. Once this substance has been internalised, it undergoes lyposomal degeneration and, as cholesterol ester, is hydrolysed to free cholesterol. Release of the free cholesterol from the lysosome regulates the cellular cholesterol content. What is this receptor?

Cardiology

Question Frequency

Alagille's syndrome (adult)	4	Chest X-ray (adult)	1
Anatomy	2	Chronic alcohol consumption	0
Angiotensin-converting enzyme		Chronic leg ulceration (adult)	1
(ACE) inhibitors	0	Chylous effusions	0
Antiarrhythmics	0	Circulatory changes in pregnancy	0
Aortic aneurysms	0	Circulatory changes on respiration	0
Aortic dissection	0	Coarctation (adult)	5
Aortic regurgitation	0	Congenital heart disease	5
Aortic stenosis	4	Congestive cardiac heart disease	0
Aortic supravalvular stenosis	0	Cornelia de Lange syndrome	0
Aortic valve stenosis	0	Coronary artery	1
Apex	0	Coronary artery disease	1
Arrhythmias	0	Cyanosis	10
Arteriovenous shunt	1	Cyanosis – central (adult)	9
Associations	1	Da Costa's syndrome	0
ATLS	0	Deep vein thrombosis	0
Atrial fibrillation (adult)	3	Dextrocardia	0
Atrial flutter (adult)	3	Diastolic murmur (adult)	2
Atrial myxomas (adult)	1	DiGeorge syndrome (adult)	4
Atrial septal defect	7	Ebstein's anomaly (adult)	3
Atrioventricular block	1	ECG	2
Atrioventricular malformations	2	ECHO	0
Atrioventricular septal defect	2	Eisenmenger's syndrome	2
Cardiac catheterisation	2	Electrical–mechanical dissociation	0
Cardiac emergencies	0	Exercise tolerance test	0
Cardiac rupture	0	Fainting	1
Cardiac sarcomere	0	Fetal circulation (adult)	5
Cardiac tumours	0	Genetics of congenital heart	
Cavernous sinus thrombosis (adult)	1	disease	2
Chest pain	0	Heart defects	2

questions

Heart failure – congestive (adult)	6	Pulmonary hypertension	0
Heart failure – refractory (adult)	6	Pulmonary valve stenosis	2
Heart sounds	6	Pulse (adult)	1
Hypertension	1	Rarities	0
Hypertension – portal	2	β-Receptors	0
Hypoplastic left heart (adult)	1	Rheumatic fever	2
Infective endocarditis	2	Shock – cardiogenic	1
Inotropes (adult)	1	Shunts	0
Ivemark syndrome	1	Sick sinus syndrome (adult)	1
Jugular venous pressure (adult)	5	Squatting	0
Keshan disease	0	ST depression	0
Left end-diastolic volume (adult)	1	Sudden death	0
Long QT syndrome	2	SVT obstruction	0
Lung cysts	0	Sympathomimetic amines	1
Lung fields	0	Syncope	0
Lung segments	0	Syndromes of congenital heart	
Middle aortic syndrome	0	disease	2
Mitral regurgitation (adult)	2	Tachycardia	4
Mitral stenosis (adult)	3	Tachycardia – supraventricular	6
Mitral valve prolapse (adult)	4	Takayasu's arteritis	0
Murmurs – innocent	4	Tetralogy of Fallot (adult)	6
Murmurs – location	0	Thoracotomy	0
Murmurs – neonatal	0	Thrills	0
Myocardial infarction	1	Thrombolysis	0
Myocarditis	0	Torsades de pointes	0
Persistent ductus arteriosus (adult)	5	Total anomalous venous drainage	
Pericardial effusions (adult)	1	(adult)	2
Pericarditis (adult)	3	Transplant	0
Pericarditis – constrictive (adult)	4	Transposition of the great arteries	0
Pericarditis – TB	0	Tricuspid atresia (adult)	2
Persistent fetal circulation	0	Truncus arteriosus	0
Pharmacology	0	Valsalva manoeuvre	0
Posture	0	Vascular ring	1
Pressure gradients	1	Ventricular failure	1
Prophylactic antibiotics	1	Ventricular septal defect (adult)	3
Pulmonary artery pressure (adult)	5	Wolff–Parkinson–White syndrome	
Pulmonary atresia	0	(adult)	6

Multiple True/False Questions

10 With respect to angiotensin-converting enzyme (ACE) inhibitors, which of the following statements are correct?

- A They are always used in the treatment of post-nephritic hypertension
- B They are contraindicated for use in pre-eclampsia
- C All have many side-effects, one of which is dysgeusia
- D They cause gout
- E Enalapril is a pro-drug that is converted to the active component enalaprat in the liver

11 Chronic alcohol consumption results in which of the following?

- A Dilated cardiomyopathy
- B Atrial flutter
- C An increased incidence of embolic and haemorrhagic stroke
- D Thiamine deficiency
- E Persistent paroxysmal tachycardia

12 Regarding aortic valve stenosis, which of the following statements is correct?

- A It is seen in 5% of children with congenital heart disease
- B It is associated with fetal phenytoin syndrome
- C It can present as sudden infant death syndrome (SIDS)
- D It is recommended for surgery if a pressure gradient of 6 mmHg is found
- E It may present clinically with an ejection click at the left lower sternal edge (LLSE) and the apex

13 With regard to atrial septal defects (ASDs) which of the following statements are true?

- A There is a female predominance
- B The murmur is caused by the flow across the septal defect
- C These defects are not associated with asplenia
- D They are not associated with polysplenia
- E Defects often present in childhood with pulmonary hypertension

14 Causes of atrial fibrillation in children include which of the following?

- A Pulmonary embolism
- B Sick sinus syndrome
- C Thyrotoxicosis
- D Atrial septal defect (ASD)
- E Mitral valve disease

15 **In atrial flutter which of the following statements are correct?**

- A There is an association with angina pectoris
- B There is an association with myocardial infarction
- C Vagal stimulation can be diagnostic
- D Quinidine increases the flutter rate
- E The condition can present with cardiac pain

Best of Five Questions

16 A 10-year-old male child with epilepsy is admitted with a heart murmur. On examination, he is hypertensive, the blood pressure greater in the proximal than the distal limbs. He has a prominent carotid pulse and a left ventricular heave on palpation. Heart sounds depict an ejection systolic murmur at the upper left sternal edge and posteriorly over the left interscapular area. An apical ejection click is audible at the apex. Palpation of the pulses shows decreased volume in the femoral arteries. The child has an abnormal chest radiograph with mild cardiomegaly and a slight abnormality of the inferior surface of the 3rd, 4th and 5th ribs. His ECG shows mild left ventricular hypertrophy.

What is the diagnosis?

- A Fracture of the 3, 4 and 5 ribs
- B Aortic stenosis
- C A bicuspid aortic valve
- D Coarctation of the aorta
- E Persistent ductus arteriosus

17 An 8-year-old girl presents with her traveller family complaining of a sore throat, fever, painful joints, a rash and abnormal movements. On examination, she looks quite miserable, with a fever of 38.4°C and an erythematous rash with raised edges. On examination, you note her to have abnormal rhythmical movements and arthralgia with associated joint swelling of the left ankle and right elbow. She has multiple painless subcutaneous nodules under her skin. On examination, she is tachycardic and hypertensive. On auscultation, there is an apical mid-diastolic murmur. Investigations show a leukocytosis with a raised C-reactive protein (CRP) level and erythrocyte sedimentation rate (ESR), and her ECG confirms a tachycardia, a prolonged PR interval and flat inverted T waves.

What is the diagnosis?

○ A Subacute bacterial endocarditis
○ B Group A β-haemolytic streptococcal throat infection ✓
○ C Systemic lupus erythematosus
○ D Juvenile chronic arthritis
○ E Rheumatic fever

18 A 6-month-old male infant is admitted with shortness of breath, oedema, cyanosis and arrhythmia. On examination, he has oedema with central cyanosis and an irregular pulse. A displaced apical beat is heard laterally, with a marked right ventricular heave and bilateral basal crackles in the chest. A chest radiograph shows gross cardiomegaly. An echocardiogram confirms mitral valve prolapse, and an ECG shows a short PR interval with a prolonged widened QRS complex and an upslurring of this complex. There is right bundle branch block and a dominant R wave in V1. What is the diagnosis?

What is the diagnosis?

○ A Mitral valve prolapse disease
○ B Type A Wolff–Parkinson–White syndrome (WPWS) ✓
○ C Type B WPWS
○ D Heart failure
○ E Myocarditis

Clinical Pharmacology

Question Frequency

Acetazolamide	0	Antifungal agents	1
Acetochlorine	1	Antiviral medication	0
Acetylation (adult)	2	Associations (adult)	2
Aciclovir	0	Asthma	1
Adenosine (adult)	1	Azathioprine	0
Administration of drug	0	β-blockers	0
Alpha blockade (adult)	1	β_2-agonists	2
Amiodarone (adult)	5	Benign intracranial	
Amiodarone – pulmonary toxicity	0	hypertension	0
Aminophylline	0	Benzodiazepines	0
Aminosalicylic acid	0	Bromocriptine	0
Amphetamines	1	Bronchospasm (adult)	2
Angiotensin 1	0	Calcium channel blockers	1
Angiotensin 2 (adult)	2	Carbimazole (adult)	1
Angiotensin-converting enzyme		Carcinogens	1
(ACE)	0	Caustic ingestion	1
Angiotensin-converting enzyme		Chloroquine	1
(ACE) inhibitors	0	Chlorpromazine	0
Antiarrhythmics	0	Ciclosporin	0
Anticonvulsant usage (adult)	2	Cimetidine	3
Anticonvulsants – carbamazepine		Cisapride	0
(adult)	2	Clinitest – false positive (adult)	2
Anticonvulsants – lamotrigine	0	Corticosteroids	1
Anticonvulsants – phenobarbitone		Cyclophosphamide	0
(adult)	3	Cytotoxic drugs	0
Anticonvulsants – phenytoin (adult)	3	Digoxin (adult)	3
Anticonvulsants – sodium		Digoxin – toxicity (adult)	2
valproate (adult)	5	Diuretics (adult)	2
Antidotes	0	Dopamine (adult)	1
Antiepileptic drugs (adult)	4	Drug-induced anaemia	0

questions

Multiple True/False Questions

19 In replacement therapy, which of the following steroids has a significant mineralocorticoid effect?

○ A Hydrocortisone
○ B Cortisone
○ C Glucocorticoid
○ D Fludrocortisone
○ E Betamethasone

20 Which of the following interactions are seen with aspirin?

○ A Increased risk of bleeding with antacids
○ B Decreased absorption with metoclopramide
○ C Reduced effect of probenicid
○ D With corticosteroids, association with an increased risk of gastrointestinal bleeding
○ E May induce an asthma attack

21 Erythromycin is the first-line drug to prevent secondary cases of which of the following diseases?

○ A Rheumatic fever
○ B Meningococcal meningitis
○ C *Haemophilus influenzae* type B
○ D Diphtheria in a non-immune patient
○ E Pertussis

22 Activated charcoal can enhance elimination following overdose with which of the following?

○ A Barbiturates
○ B Carbamazepine
○ C Dapsone
○ D Quinine
○ E Theophylline

23 Which of the following can be treated by the use of a specific antidote?

○ A Pethidine
○ B Paracetamol
○ C Ferrous sulphate
○ D Aspirin
○ E Lithium

questions

24 Of the following five complications, which one is not associated with NSAID usage?

○ A Renal papillary necrosis
○ B Hyperkalaemia
○ C Gastritis
○ D Internal bleeding
○ E Nephrotic syndrome

Best of Five Questions

25 This drug is a class 3 antiarrhythmic drug. It is a vasodilator of both the peripheral and the central circulation, and is a negative chronotrope. It has a half-life of 7–8 weeks and needs a loading dose. It acts to prolong the action potential in the refractory period. It also prolongs the QT and QRS complexes and is a sodium channel blocker. It directly decreases the automaticity of the sinus and the autonomic nervous system, and has α- and β-blocking properties.

What is this drug?

○ A Digoxin
○ B Amiodarone
○ C Adenosine
○ D Flecainide
○ E Atropine

26 This antiepileptic medication is used to enhance the action of γ-aminobutyric acid, which is a major inhibitory neurotransmitter. It is used in absence attacks, temporal lobe epilepsy and myoclonic-type epilepsy. It inhibits liver enzymes and may enhance the function of other antiepileptic agents such as phenytoin, causing toxicity.

What is this medication?

○ A Sodium valproate
○ B Phenytoin
○ C Vigabatrin
○ D Topiramate
○ E Carbamazepine

27 A teenager presents unconscious in the A&E department. Her parents give a history that she had been drinking the night before. During the night, she complained of a high fever and sweating with severe abdominal pain. She also intermittently complained of dizziness, tinnitus and deafness. The girl became very irritable and therefore went to bed thinking that this was due to alcohol toxicity. Next morning, she was found unconscious. Investigations have revealed the following results: sodium 130 mmol/l, potassium 2.9 mmol/l, urea 9.4 mmol/l, creatinine 115 μmol/l, hypoprothrombinaemia and a normal bleeding time on clotting analysis, blood glucose 2.1 mmol/l, urinalysis test positive and blood gases showing a compensated metabolic acidosis. She has also presented with bruising.

What is the diagnosis?

- ○ A Codeine phosphate toxicity
- ○ B Paracetamol toxicity
- ○ C Salicylate toxicity
- ○ D Alcohol toxicity
- ○ E Ibuprofen toxicity

questions

Dermatology

Question Frequency

Acanthosis nigrans	0	Epidermal naevi	1
Acne	1	Epidermolysis bullosa	1
Acrodermatitis enteropathica	1	Erythema marginatum	1
Adenoma sebaceum	1	Erythema multiforme	5
Albinism	1	Erythema neonatorum	0
Alopecia (adult)	2	Erythema nodosum	3
Anaphylactoid purpura	1	Erythematous maculopapular rash	
Angiokeratoma corporis diffusum	1	(adult)	1
Anhidrotic ectodermal dysplasia	1	Fragile skin (adult)	1
Arsenic poisoning	0	Fungal infections	0
Basal cell carcinomas	1	Gianotti–Crosti syndrome	1
Birth mark	1	Granuloma annulare	1
Blistering	1	Haemangioma – cavernous	1
Blisters, vesicles, bullae	0	Haemangiomas	1
Bullous eruption	1	Haemorrhages of the skin	0
Café au lait spots	1	Hair abnormalities	0
Candidiasis	1	Hand, foot and mouth infection	1
Cephalohaematoma	1	Herpes gestationis	1
Collodion baby (adult)	2	Herpes infection skin	0
Congenital teeth	1	Hirsutism	1
Cutis marmorata	1	Hyperpigmentation	0
Dermatitis	2	Hypertrichosis	1
Dermatitis artefacta	1	Hypomelanosis of Ito	0
Dermatological treatments	0	Hypopigmentation	1
Dermatophyte lesions	1	Ichthymoses	1
Diabetic lesions (adult)	2	Impetigo	1
Drug-induced rashes	0	Incontinentia pigmenti	3
Eczema	2	Infantile acne	0
Ehlers–Danlos syndrome	0	Infection skin	0

questions

Keloid	0	Port wine stain	1
Kerion	1	Pruritic rashes (adult)	1
Klippel–Trenaunay syndrome	1	*Pseudomonas*	1
Koebner phenomenon	1	Psoriasis	4
LCH	1	Purpuric skin lesions	1
Lichen planus	1	Pyoderma gangrenosum	0
Lichen sclerosus et atrophicus	1	Pyogenic granuloma	0
Lichen striatus	1	Rash – itchy, widespread (adult)	2
Lyell's disease	1	Scabies	1
Malignant melanoma	0	Scarlet fever	1
Malignant skin lesions	1	Scarring (adult)	1
Manifestations of systemic disease (adult)	1	Sebaceous naevus	0
		Seborrheic dermatitis	1
Mastocytosis	0	Skin immunology	0
Melatonin	1	Skin tests (adult)	1
Molluscum contagiosum	1	Skin tumours	1
Mongolian blue spot	2	Staphylococcal scalded skin syndrome	1
Morphea	0		
Naevi	1	Stevens Johnson syndrome	1
Nail abnormalities	0	Syphilis	1
Nail changes	2	Thrombocytopenic purpura	0
Nail pitting	2	Tinea	2
Nappy rash	1	Tinea capitis (adult)	3
Neurofibromatosis	1	Toxic epidermal necrolysis	1
Orogenital ulceration	1	Toxic shock syndrome	1
Palms and soles	0	Trichotillomania	1
Paraneoplastic syndromes	0	Urticaria	2
Pemphigoid	1	Variceal haemorrhage	0
Pemphigus	1	Vascular malformations	0
Peutz–Jeghers syndrome	1	Vasculitides	0
Photosensitivity drugs	1	Viral xanthemata	1
Photosensitivity rashes (adult)	5	Vitiligo	0
Pigmentation	1	Waardenburg's syndrome	0
Pityriasis lichenoides	1	Warts	1
Pityriasis rosea	2	Xeroderma pigmentosa	0
Pityriasis versicolor	2		
Poikiloderma atrophicans vasculare	0		

Best of Five Questions

28 A 6-year-old girl presents with a fine, hyperpigmented, streaky whorl rash over her left thigh and a wart-like lesion. She has suffered from seizures since she was 3 years of age, and she has complained of stubborn warts in the past. Her mother has had two in utero stillbirths but no other family history of note. On examination, crops of small vesicles are found on the ventral surface of the girl's left wrist. She has a mild scoliosis but a normal gait, thin wiry hair and peg-shaped teeth. Cardiovascular, respiratory and abdominal examination is unremarkable. Her Ruth Griffiths score has shown her to have a reduced subquotient in the categories of social skills, language and hearing, and performance. A skin biopsy confirms a large number of intradermal eosinophils but no inflammatory cells.

What is the cause of this girl's hyperkeratotic hypermelanotic lesion?

- ○ A Herpes simplex infection
- ○ B Bullous impetigo
- ○ C Erythema bullosa
- ○ D Incontinentia pigmenti
- ○ E Warts

29 A 4-year-old boy is found by the school nurse to have an annular erythematous scaly lesion on his left forearm. He has been playing with his pet dog over the weekend. This lesion is pruritic in nature and on palpation has a raised circumferential edge with a clear, flat centre. Skin scrapings are sent to the laboratory for analysis, and the boy is treated with antifungal medication for his skin, hair and nails.

What is this diagnosis?

- ○ A Tinea versicolor
- ○ B Tinea capitis
- ○ C Tinea corporis
- ○ D Discoid psoriasis
- ○ E Diabeticorum annulare

Extended Matching Question

30 Theme: Rashes

A Chronic idiopathic urticaria
B Hereditary angioneurotic oedema
C Erythema multiforme
D Stevens–Johnson syndrome
E Erythema nodosum
F Insect bite
G Scalded skin syndrome
H Erysipelas
I Kawasaki's disease
J Slapped cheek syndrome

Match the following three clinical scenarios to one of the clinical diagnoses above.

○ 1 A 4-year-old girl presents to the A&E department with a 3-day history of fever (38.4°C), a prodromal illness, concurrent malaise and arthralgia. She has recently been commenced on penicillin for a sore throat. On examination, she has characteristic target lesions, which are macular-papular on palpation, with a surrounding purplish hue and a central erythematous white wheal. These heliotrope papules involve the hands, feet and extensor surfaces. What is the diagnosis?

○ 2 A 13-year-old girl recently returned from a snorkelling holiday in Malta. She presents acutely with a 3-day history of high fever, malaise, purulent conjunctivitis, arthralgia and photophobia. On examination, she is unwell, with mucositis and inflamed conjunctivae. She has swelling of both knees and the left ankle, and a marked non-desquamating rash. Investigations confirm a right lower lobe pneumonia, hypercalcaemia, hyponatraemia, a leukocytosis, and a raised C-reactive (CRP) level of 240. This episode resolved with frequent benzydamine hydrochloride (Difflam) spray, chlorhexidine mouthwashes and a 6-week course of intravenous ceftriaxone, aciclovir and clarithromycin, with hydrocortisone support. The girl's ophthalmic lesions were managed with protective eye care. What is the diagnosis?

○ 3 An 8-year-old girl presents with a 2-year history of an erythematous, urticarial, pruritic rash associated with episodes of stress, heat, cold baths and trauma. On examination, she appears fit and well with no evidence of hay fever, rhinitis, mucosal pleats, asthma or urticarial rash. All investigations are unremarkable, including a moderately low C1 esterase inhibitor level. The girl's symptoms resolve with chlorpheniramine for acute episodes of urticaria.

Development

Question Frequency

Deafness	4	Primitive reflexes (adult)	3
Developmental regression	3	Reading delay	2
Drawing	3	Screening	2
Dubowitz score	1	Screening programme (adult)	2
Figures	3	Speech delay	2
Hearing	2	Speech discrimination test	1
Language delay	3	Vision	1

Multiple True/False Questions

31 What is this girl's developmental age with respect to her drawing fine motor skills?

A girl presents with dyspraxia. At mainstream school, they have noticed that she has difficulty with dressing, undressing, doing up her buttons and tying her shoelaces. She holds a pencil with a mature pincer grasp in her right hand. She is able to copy a horizontal line, vertical line, circle, ladder, square, triangle and slanted rectangle, but she has difficulty copying a diamond. She can draw her house, her father and a ladder to stage II in all categories, and is able to write her first name but not her surname.

- ○ A 5 years
- ○ B 5.5 years
- ○ C 6 years
- ○ D 6.5 years
- ○ E 7 years

32 Which one of the following tests would *not* be suitable for a girl of this age?

A 6-month-old baby girl is referred to the audiologist for an assessment of hearing. At the 6-week check, the GP noted that she was not responding to surrounding noises. Two to three months later, she did not appear to have any interest in toys or people.

- ○ A Startle test
- ○ B Oto-acoustic emission test
- ○ C Brainstem-evoked auditory responses
- ○ D Distraction test
- ○ E Pure tone audiometry

33 Normal motor development at 3 months includes which of the following?

- ○ A Pulling to sit, with head lag
- ○ B Tonic neck reflex posture with the head to one side
- ○ C Attempts to crawl
- ○ D Finger play with the hands open and brought together
- ○ E Sitting with support

34 By 2 years, a child should be able to do which of the following?

- ○ A Pull and push large wheeled toys and squat to play with toys on the floor
- ○ B Climb on to the furniture
- ○ C Run on tiptoe

○ D Ride a tricycle and turn wide corners
○ E Stand on one leg for 3–5 seconds
○ F Walk along a dotted line
○ G Crawl downstairs

35 Normal hearing and speech at 3 months of age reveal themselves by which of the following?

○ A Crying when uncomfortable and annoyed
○ B Vocalising delightedly when spoken to
○ C Babbling loudly and tunefully with repetitive strings of syllables, eg ba-ba
○ D Imitating adults' playful vocalisations
○ E Understanding the word 'no'

36 By 18 months of age, which of the following gross motor skills should have been acquired?

○ A Propelling a tricycle forwards by pushing with the feet on the floor
○ B Throwing a small ball overhand without falling
○ C Walking into a large ball when trying to kick it
○ D Jumping with two feet together from a low step
○ E Standing on tiptoe if shown

Best of Five Questions

37 A 2-year-old Somali boy has attended a day nursery for the first time since arriving in the UK. The teacher has found that the boy plays very much on his own and appears very shy. He does not seem to react to verbal communication, loud sounds or songs sung around him. He appears to be a very happy child who gives good eye contact; once engagement has been sought, he shows good interactive play. He sleeps for 6–7 hours during the day as well as 12 hours at night. His four siblings suffer from otitis media, and his brother has been found eating dirt and biting the paint off the side of the house. Investigations on the boy show normal electrolyte, C-reactive protein, full blood count and full septic screen readings. Urine and serum toxicology prove negative. The only abnormality is a mildly raised thyroid-stimulating hormone level. An audiology review reports that he has bilateral sensorineural deafness.

What is a possible diagnosis for this boy?

○ A Lead encephalopathy
○ B Hypothyroidism
○ C Pendred's syndrome
○ D Waardenburg's syndrome
○ E Chronic suppurative otitis media

38 An infant presents to the GP for her routine check. During a developmental assessment, she is able to transfer a cube from her left to her right hand, obtain a raisin in a mature pincer grasp and gain much excitement when placed in a forward or downward parachute position. She no longer has a rooting, grasp or startle reflex, and her symmetrical Moro reflex has disappeared. The infant continuously presents items to her mouth and sucks her fingers. She has a positive Babinski sign but a negative asymmetrical tonic chronic reflex.

What developmental age is this girl?

○ A 2 months
○ B 3 months
○ C 8 months
○ D 12 months
○ E 18 months

Extended Matching Questions

39 Theme: Developmental regression

A Hypothyroidism
B Batten disease
C Aminoaciduria disorder
D Human immunodeficiency virus (HIV) encephalopathy
E Peroxisomal disorders
F Lead encephalopathy
G Subacute sclerosing panencephalopathy
H Spieler–Mayer–Schrögen syndrome
I Leigh's encephalopathy
J Hydrocephalus secondary to a medulloblastoma

Three children present to the child development centre for assessment of developmental regression. The diagnoses listed above are possible causes for developmental regression. Match the three clinical scenarios to one diagnosis from the diagnostic suggestions above.

○ 1 A 3-year-old boy and his parents review a hospice. He presented previously with myoclonic jerks, optic atrophy and progressive dementia. His parents have found it increasingly difficult to control his myoclonic jerks and he is becoming increasingly agitated, requiring sedation. A bone marrow sample found lipofuscin in his marrow cells. What is his diagnosis?

○ 2 A 14-year-old Iranian girl presents with a 6-month history of developmental regression. She has regressed in all categories of her development and now wears nappies both day and night. She has ten words in her own language and appears unable to communicate. There is no previous medical history to note. She is unvaccinated. She has had all the usual childhood rashes. On clinical examination, she is well. Her Griffiths mental scale scoring portrays her subquotient results as follows: gross motor 8.5 months, social skills 12 months, language and hearing 14 months, and hand and eye coordination 18 months; she was unable to carry out the performance tasks. What is the most likely cause of this girl's developmental regression?

○ 3 An 8-year-old girl presents with a 12-month history of early morning headaches with associated nausea and vomiting before breakfast. She is otherwise fit and well. Her friends have noticed that she does not participate in lunchtime meals as she used to. On clinical examination, she is found to have increased reflexes and clonus on the right side. On ophthalmic examination, there is papilloedema of the left eye. What is her diagnosis?

40 Theme: Speech delay

    A Tongue-tie
    B Down's syndrome
    C Secretory otitis media
    D Duchenne muscular dystrophy
    E Autism
    F Bilingual family
    G Emotional deprivation
    H Hypothyroidism
    I Phenylketonuria
    J Meningitis

The above are common causes of speech delay. Match a diagnosis for each of the three clinical scenarios to the list above.

○ 1 A 3-year-old Somali girl is referred for poor hearing and an assessment for possible secretory otitis media. She speaks only 10–20 words and has basic sentence construction. None of her seven siblings has a hearing problem. On examination, she is quiet and withdrawn, slightly dishevelled but interacting well with other children. What is the cause of her speech and language delay?

2 A 3½-year-old boy is brought to the GP with naughty behaviour. He does not carry out tasks asked of him and does not listen to what he is told. Over the winter period, he has had recurrent febrile coryzal illnesses but has otherwise remained well. He is found to have conductive hearing loss. What is his diagnosis?

3 A blond, blue-eyed, 4½-year-old girl presents to the child development centre for a developmental assessment. Her previous medical history is unremarkable, with a normal neonatal period and a normal Guthrie test. Her elder brother has dyslexia and dyspraxia. She has a poor attention span with limited listening skills. She does not engage fully with the assessor and gives poor eye contact. The girl is found to have marked expressive and receptive language delay, with poor social skills; the score in all categories is reduced due to her severely impaired literacy and numeracy skills. On examination, she has poor speech, echolalia and repetitive movements, and is easily distracted. What is her diagnosis?

Embryology

Question Frequency

Associations	0	Male	3
Brachial arches	3	Pituitary gland	0
Cardiogenesis	0	Renal	0
Cardiovascular system	0	Skin and hair	0
Central nervous system	0	Spinal cord	0
Endocrine	1	Endoderm	3
Eye	0	Fetomaternal circulation	2
Gastrointestinal tract	0	Gametogenesis	2
Genital system	0	Intestinal development	0
Lungs	3		

Multiple True/False Questions

41 With regard to the fetomaternal circulation, which of the following five statements is *incorrect*?

○ A Development of the uteroplacental circulation commences at 72 days and is fully established within the 7th week after fertilisation

○ B Trophoblastic lacunae develop within the syncytiotrophoblast

○ C Maternal capillaries within this area expand to form maternal sinusoids

○ D Extra-embryonic mesoderm grows and extends into the primary stem villi to become secondary villi

○ E The placenta produces steroid hormones and prostaglandins

42 Of the following five pharyngeal pouches, which is responsible for the development of the thymus?

○ A First pouch

○ B Second pouch

○ C Third pouch

○ D Fourth pouch

○ E Fifth pouch

Extended Matching Questions

43 Theme: Branchial arches

A First arch – anterior two-thirds of the tongue

B Second arch

C Third arch – posterior third of the tongue

D Fourth arch – small part of the dorsum of the tongue

E First pouch – tympanic cavity and auditory tube

F Second pouch – tongue and palatine tonsils

G Third pouch – thymus and inferior parathyroid gland

H Fourth pouch – superior parathyroid gland (C cells)

I First pharyngeal cleft – external auditory meatus

J All of the above

The derivative anatomy of the pharyngeal arches, pouches and clefts is required in order to understand various abnormalities. Match the abnormalities in the three scenarios given below to the branchial arches above.

○ 1 Abnormalities of the thyroid gland are associated with an abnormality of two of the above branchial arches. Which two?

○ 2 A child presents to the clinic with Pierre Robin sequence, and the parent asks which branchial arch abnormality is associated with this syndrome. What is your suggestion to her?

○ 3 A child presents to the clinic with 22q11 microdeletion (DiGeorge) syndrome and you are advising the parents why this child presents with possible immune deficiency and hypocalcaemia. A possible explanation is an abnormality of which of the above pharyngeal pouches?

44 Theme: Impaired fetal lung development

A Cardiothoracic dystrophy
B Duchenne muscular dystrophy
C Infant of an insulin-dependent diabetic mother
D Potter's syndrome
E Bronchiolitis
F Jeune's syndrome (asphyxiating thoracic dystrophy)
G Facioscapulohumeral dystrophy
H Dystrophia myotonia
I Pickwickian syndrome
J Kartagener's syndrome

Impaired fetal lung development is seen in many conditions. For the ten disorders above, match a possible diagnosis to one of the three scenarios given below.

○ 1 You attend the urgent delivery of a 38-week gestation male infant with severe difficulty breathing. After full resuscitation, he is intubated, ventilated and managed on the neonatal intensive care unit. On examination, he is found to be dysmorphic with maxillary hyperplasia, micrognathia and a small chest. Further investigations show him to have posterior urethral valves. What is his diagnosis?

○ 2 You review a 4-year-old girl in the orthopaedic clinic who has recently had cartilage inserted into her anterior mediastinum. She was born at 32 weeks' gestation and was intubated and ventilated at birth due to difficulty breathing. She was found to have severe lung hypoplasia and has subsequently required the insertion of cartilage to her sternum to accommodate the increase in growth. What is her diagnosis?

○ 3 You are asked to review an intubated and ventilated male child in intensive care who is hypotonic and lying in a frog-like position. Important antenatal history includes polyhydramnios. Interestingly, when you shake the mother's hand she is unable to release her grip, and when asked to close her eyes she is unable to open them effectively. What is his diagnosis?

45 Theme: Development of the genitalia

A Coelomic epithelium
B Mesenchymal cells
C Sertoli cells
D Allantois
E Urachus
F Mesonephros
G Paramesonephric duct
H Mesonephric duct
I Develop in the 9th thoracic level
J Develop in the 10th thoracic level

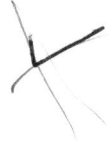

For the three statements below, which items in the above list are correct?

○○○ 1 Which **three** items relate to the development of the *male* genitalia?

○○ 2 Which **two** items relate to the development of the *female* genitalia?

○○○○ 3 Which **four** items relate to the development of *both* male and female genitalia?

Emergency Medicine

Question Frequency

Abdominal pain	2	Hyperglycaemia	6
Acute deafness	3	Hypertension	2
Allergy	12	Hypoglycaemia	5
Arrhythmias	0	Infantile seizures	4
Asthma	12	Infective endocarditis	2
ATLS	0	Intestinal obstruction	1
Atrioventricular block	1	Intussusception	3
Bleeding	7	Joint pain	1
Bruising	1	Malignancy risks	1
Burns	12	Meningitis	3
Cardiac emergencies	0	Migraine	4
Cardiac rupture	0	Myocardial infarction	1
Cardiogenic shock	1	Neonatal fits	3
Chest pain	0	Oculogyric crisis	1
Congestive cardiac heart disease	0	Osteomyelitis	0
Cyanosis	10	Pneumonia	3
Dehydration	6	Salt-losing crisis	2
Diarrhoea	9	Scrotal swelling	1
Drug overdose	6	Self-induced harm	2
Drug-induced rashes	0	Sickle cell crisis	2
Electrical–mechanical dissociation	0	Subarachnoid haemorrhage	2
Epilepsy	6	Suicide	0
Fainting	1	Supraventricular tachycardia	6
Floppy infant	1	Synovial fluid	1
Fluid resuscitation	5	Trauma	10
Fractures	3	Vaccine contraindications	2
Gastroenteritis	2	Valsalva manoeuvre	6
Head injury	3	Volvulus	1
Headache	6	Vomiting	6
Heart failure	6	Whooping cough	4
Hemiplegia	2		

Multiple True/False Questions

46 For the emergency treatment of anaphylaxis

○ A   the first step is the administration of chlorpheniramine
○ B   the administration of intravenous epinephrine is mandatory
○ C   the dosage of epinephrine should be 0.1 ml/kg of 1:1000 in all cases
○ D   the dose of epinephrine should be repeated after 10 minutes if there is no clinical improvement
○ E   as evidenced by bronchospasm without hypotension, inhaled salbutamol must be used in place of adrenaline

47 Which of the following are true for the use of adrenaline in resuscitation?

○ A   It may be administered at a dosage of 10 mg/kg intravenously or i.o.
○ B   It should not be given in conjunction with sodium bicarbonate
○ C   It may be given at a higher dose intravenously or i.o. in the case of cardiorespiratory arrest if the cause is thought to be circulatory collapse
○ D   It can be used in the treatment of symptomatic bradycardia
○ E   It makes ventricular fibrillation more likely to respond to DC defibrillation

48 Which of the following drugs can be given via the endotracheal route as they are lipid soluble?

○ A   Calcium chloride
○ B   Sodium bicarbonate
○ C   Lidocaine (lignocaine)
○ D   Epinephrine (adrenaline)
○ E   Naloxone

Endocrinology

Question Frequency

questions

Multiple True/False Questions

49 Regarding congenital adrenal hyperplasia (CAH), which of the following statements are correct?

○ A The commonest type is 21-hydroxylase deficiency
○ B If the condition is caused by classic 21-hydroxylase deficiency, virilisation of the female is seen
○ C If it results from 11β-hydroxylase, virilisation is seen in the female
○ D It can present with a high urinary sodium level and dehydration
○ E If due to 3β-hydroxysteroid dehyrogenase deficiency, the neonate can present with clitoromegaly

50 Which of the following are endocrine causes of hypertension?

○ A Phaeochromocytoma
○ B Hyperaldosteronism
○ C Diabetes mellitus
○ D Congenital adrenal hyperplasia due to 3β-hydroxysteroid dehydrogenase deficiency
○ E Cushing's syndrome

Best of Five Questions

51 You review a 12-year-old boy for a pubertal assessment. His results are as follows:

Genital stage:
- **Testes – 4–5 ml testicular enlargement**
- **Scrotum – thin with red pigment, rugosity and penile lengthening and widening**
- **Pubic hair – developed**
- **Axillary hair – developed**
- **Peak height velocity – has not yet reached his peak height velocity**

Which of the following pubertal developmental stages fits the above scenario?

○ A Genital stage 1, pubic stage 2, axillary stage 2, peak height velocity not reached
○ B Genital stage 2, pubic stage 2, axillary stage 2, peak height velocity not reached
○ C Genital stage 3, pubic stage 4, axillary stage 2, peak height velocity not reached
○ D Genital stage 4, pubic stage 4, axillary stage 3, peak height velocity not reached
○ E Genital stage 5, pubic stage 5, axillary stage 3, peak height velocity reached

52 A 6-year-old female infant attends with a buttock swelling. On examination, she is afebrile with normal observations. There is a slightly discolored raised swelling of the left buttock, not crossing the midline, and with no neurocutaneous markers. Investigations show a normal full blood count and C-reactive protein level, raised gonadotrophin-releasing hormone, raised follicle-stimulating hormone, a luteinising hormone level of over 10, abnormal pituitary and adrenal function, a raised oestradiol level, an advanced bone age on X-ray, a normal magnetic resonance imaging scan of the brain and, on ultrasonography, a mass containing cysts and undefined tissue. Pelvic ultrasound is normal. The girl's pubertal assessment states that she has breast stage 4, pubic hair stage 4, axillary hair stage 3, menarche 0 and peak height velocity reached with breast stage 3. Which of the following diagnoses is most plausible?

Which diagnosis fits the following clinical picture?

- A Ovarian carcinoma
- B Neurofibromatosis
- C Teratoma
- D Piloma
- E Buttock abscess

53 A 15-year-old male presents with short stature and a delayed pubertal growth spurt. Over the past 6 months, he has suffered with intermittent headaches, tiredness and weight gain. On enquiry, his father was also short as a teenager and there is no family history of any endocrine abnormality. On examination, the boy is on the 9th centile for height, with delayed adrenarche and gonadarche. Cardiovascular, respiratory, abdominal and neurological examinations are unremarkable. Investigations show that thyroid function tests, gonadotrophin-releasing hormone stimulation tests, human chorionic gonadotrophin testosterone stimulation test, lateral skull X-ray and magnetic resonance imaging of the brain are all normal. He shows decreased height velocity and a decrease in his bone age. Ophthalmic examination is unremarkable.

The following five diagnoses may cause delayed puberty; which one is consistent with this clinical picture?

- A Craniopharyngioma
- B Gymnastics fanatic
- C Constitutional physiological delay of growth
- D Hypothyroidism
- E Cyproterone acetate intoxication

questions

54 A 15-year-old boy presents with a history of fainting. At birth, he had normal centiles but a raised occipitofrontal circumference with a normal magnetic resonance imaging (MRI) scan. On observation, he has a male habitus, is above the 75th centile for height, is below the 50th centile for weight and has an occipitofrontal circumference below the 50th centile, with pectus excavatum and pectus carinatum. He has marked flexibility of the joints, arachnoidactyly and a high-arched palate. Ophthalmoscopy confirms ectopia lentis. On examination, the boy has a soft 2/6 ejection systolic murmur at the upper right second intercostal space, radiating to the carotid arteries. Blood pressure is normal. Respiratory, abdominal and neurological examinations are unremarkable. Investigations show a dilated aorta. His cerebral MRI scan, magnetic resonance angiography (MRA), ECG and blood tests are unremarkable.

What is the diagnosis in the above scenario?

- ○ A Familial tall stature
- ○ B Pituitary gigantism
- ○ C Hyperthyroidism
- ○ D Homocystinuria
- ○ E Marfan's syndrome

Extended Matching Questions

55 Theme: Obesity

- A Laurence–Moon–Biedl syndrome
- B Familial obesity
- C Exogenous obesity
- D Hydrocephalus
- E Alström syndrome
- F Pickwickian syndrome
- G Constitutional obesity
- H Prader–Willi syndrome
- I Morgary–Stewart–Morel syndrome
- J Organic endocrinal obesity

The above are disorders associated with obesity. Match the three clinical scenarios to one of the diagnoses listed above.

- ○ 1 You review an obese child with learning difficulties. He suffers from hypertension. On examination, you find a boy with short stature, hypogonadism, hypotonia and polydactyly. He wears glasses for reading. The ophthalmic examination is unremarkable. What is the diagnosis?

2 You review a 6-year-old boy with moderate learning difficulties. The nurse is concerned as he has had a rapid increase in weight and a deterioration in his eyesight. You find a small, obese boy who is wearing glasses for reading. On examination, he has hypogonadism and polydactyly. Ophthalmic examination confirms retinitis pigmentosa.

3 You review an intelligent 14-year-old boy who is complaining of tall stature and obesity. His previous medical history includes early weaning onto SMA Gold formula, and he has subsequently suffered from poor diet and behavioural concerns at school. He dislikes exercise. He progressed into puberty 6 months earlier than his classmates. The only abnormal investigation is an advanced bone age. His parents would like an answer for his obesity. What is the diagnosis?

56 Theme: Short stature

A Familial short stature
B Constitutional delay of growth and puberty
C Insulin-dependent diabetes mellitus
D Spondylo-epiphyseal dysplasia
E Hypochondroplasia
F Cerebral space-occupying lesion
G Growth hormone deficiency and insufficiency
H Mauriac's syndrome
I Cockayne's syndrome
J Laron syndrome

The above ten diagnosis all present with short stature. Match the following three clinical scenarios to a defined diagnosis above.

1 A 15-year-old boy presents with short stature. On examination, his height is less than the 0.4th centile, his weight is on the 75th centile and his head circumference is on the 50th centile. He appears to have normal facies with a normal IQ, examination and pubertal status. All investigations are normal. What is the underlying diagnosis?

2 A 15-year-old boy presents with a 1-year history of chronic headache and abdominal pain with associated lethargy. He has had intermittent streaks of blood in his stools. There is a family history of short stature and obesity. Otherwise, he is a scrum-half in the school rugby team and has a good appetite. On examination, the boy is obese and his height is below the 9th centile. Cardiovascular, respiratory, abdominal, neurological and ophthalmic examination is entirely unremarkable. His pubertal status is stage 1. Investigations are normal. In plotting his centiles, he has a decreased height velocity, and his radiograph confirms a decrease in bone age. What is the underlying diagnosis?

○ 3 You review a child with a skeletal dysplasia. On examination, you find a very small child with a short trunk length and normal limb lengths on radiography. What may the underlying diagnosis be?

ENT

Question Frequency

Acute otitis media	2	Hearing loss – sensorineural	3
Adenotonsillectomy	1	Periauricular skin tag	2
Audiometry	2	Retropharyngeal abscess	1
Audiometry – pure tone	2	Sinusitis	0
Cleft lip and palate	3	Sternocleidomastoid	1
Deafness	1	Tonsillar exudate	2
Deafness – congenital	1	Torticollis	1
Deafness – inherited	1	Tracheostomy	0
Distraction tests	2	Tympanogram	3
Hearing loss – conductive	3	Vocal cord dysfunction	1

Multiple True/False Question

57 What is the cause of this child's hearing deficit?

A 2½-year-old boy presents with expressive and receptive speech and language delay. He has a cleft palate abnormality. His previous medical history includes prematurity (36/40 gestation), recurrent viral illnesses during the winter months and chicken pox. Both parents are smokers. On examination, the child is afebrile, fit and well with mild submandibular lymphadenopathy. He appears unkempt but otherwise happy and gives good eye contact. Cardiovascular, respiratory and abdominal examination is unremarkable. An audiology assessment shows conductive hearing loss.

- ○ A Neglect
- ○ B Eustachian tube abnormality
- ○ C Chronic suppurative otitis media
- ○ D Congenital deafness
- ○ E Mastoiditis

Best of Five Question

58 You review a male neonate, less than 4 hours old, who presents with marked respiratory difficulty. On examination, he is dysmorphic with low-set ears, mandibular hypoplasia, micrognathia and a cleft lip and palate. He appears to be tachypnoeic and tachycardic, with a venous saturation of 82% in air. Cardiovascular and abdominal examination is unremarkable. On observation of the baby's chest, a marked tracheal tug and subcostal recession are noted, along with poor air entry bilaterally.

1 *Which would be the most appropriate treatment after giving facial oxygen?*

- ○ A External chest compression
- ○ B Bag and mask ventilation
- ○ C Nasopharyngeal intubation
- ○ D Endotracheal intubation
- ○ E Cricothyroidectomy

2   *Which of the following five associated problems is of most concern?*

○ A Difficulty breastfeeding
○ B Respiratory disease
○ C Malocclusion of the teeth later in life
○ D Hearing loss
○ E Chronic obstructive apnoea

3   *What is the most likely diagnosis?*

○ A Patau's syndrome
○ B Edwards' syndrome
○ C Pierre Robin sequence
○ D Treacher Collins syndrome
○ E Cockayne syndrome

Extended Matching Question

59 Theme: Hearing deficit

A Alport's syndrome
B Gentamicin toxicity
C Down's syndrome
D Allergic rhinitis
E Serous otitis media
F Pendred's syndrome
G Turner's syndrome
H Immunodeficiency
I   Kernicterus
J   CHARGE syndrome

Consider the following clinical situations

1 The result of a pure tone audiogram is given to the senior house officer for discussion. There is a wide discrepancy of the left ear, with the audiogram displaying a large air–bone gap. There appears to be a tone deficit of –30 decibels. Which three of the above may cause this audiogram result?

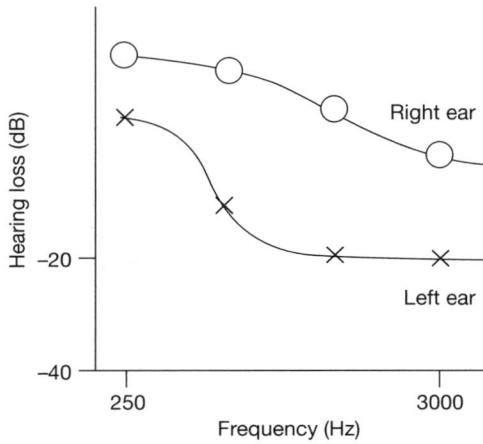

2 The senior house officer is presented with a second pure tone audiogram result for discussion. This shows a marked decrease in tone of the order of –80 decibels. No air–bone gap is noted. Which five of the above may cause this audiogram result?

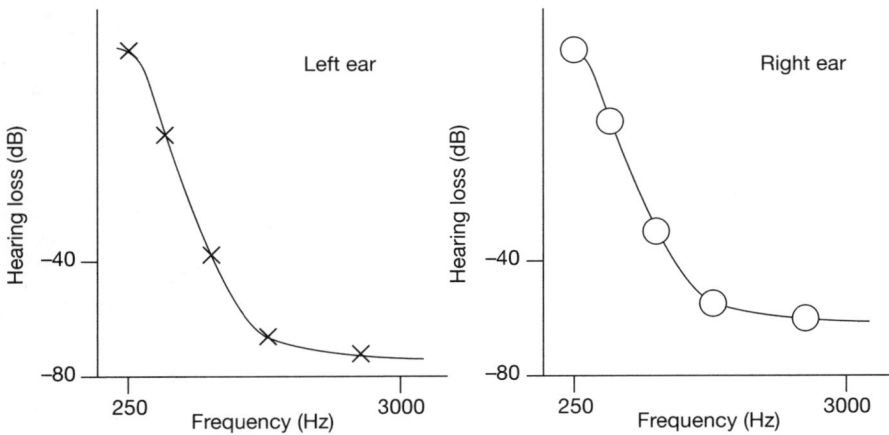

3 The senior house officer is presented with a third pure tone audiogram for discussion. This audiogram shows a mixed air–bone gap deficit and a hearing loss of the order of –70 decibels. Which three of the above may cause this audiogram result?

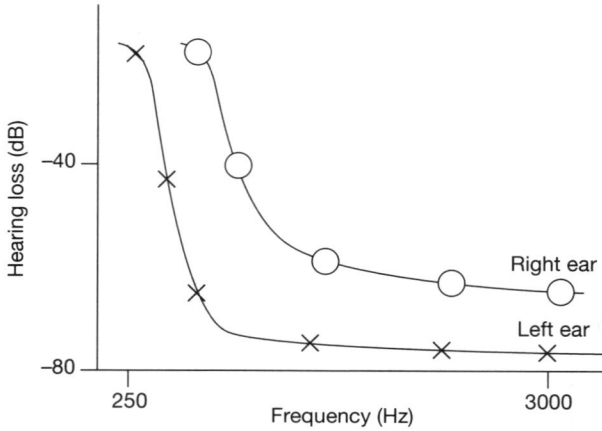

Gastroenterology

Question Frequency

Abdominal masses	0	Biliary system	3
Abdominal pain – anaemia	1	Blind loop syndrome	1
Abdominal pain – central nervous system features	1	Breast milk	5
		Bruising	1
Abdominal pain – hyponatraemia	1	Calories	1
Abdominal pain – recurrent	2	Carbohydrate digestion	0
Abdominal scars	1	Carbohydrate intolerance	0
Abetalipoproteinaemia	4	Cholestasis – neonatal	1
Acanthocytosis	2	Chronic fatigue sydrome	1
Achlorhydria (adult)	2	Coeliac disease (adult)	10
Acrodermatitis enteropathica	2	Colitis	1
Adenocarcinoma of colon	2	Colonic pseudo-obstruction	0
AIDS	0	Colorectal cancer	1
Amoebic liver abcess (adult)	1	Colostrum	0
Anatomy	0	Congenital microvillous atrophy	1
Anorectal atresia	1	Constipation	1
Antibiotics	1	Cow's milk intolerance (paed)	6
Anus	1	Cow's milk intolerance (adult)	6
Aphthous ulcers	1	Cystic fibrosis	1
Appendicitis	5	Dehydration	6
Ascites	1	Dental	0
Associations (adult)	3	Diarrhoea	4
Bacterial overgrowth	0	Diarrhoea – bloody (adult)	9
Barium swallow	1	Diarrhoea – chloride losing	2
Barrett's oesophagitis (adult)	2	Diarrhoea – protracted	3
Bezoars	1	Diarrhoea – toddler	3
Biliary atresia – extrahepatic (adult)	4	Duodenal stenosis/atresia	1
		Duodenal ulcers (adult)	2
Biliary colic	1	Duplication cysts	1

questions

Electrolyte concentration	0	Haemorrhage (adult)	2
Enteral feeds	0	*Helicobacter pylori* (adult)	9
Enteropathy	1	Hepatic adenoma	1
Enteropathy – protein losing	2	Hepatitis	3
Exophthalmos	2	Hepatitis – A	3
Faecal-oral route investigations	1	Hepatitis – autoimmune	1
Failure to thrive	1	Hepatitis – B (adult)	4
Familial adenomatous polyposis		Hepatitis – B, immunisation	1
(adult)	2	Hepatitis – C (adult)	5
Fatty acids	0	Hepatitis – chronic	3
Fatty liver	0	Hepatitis – chronic active	1
Fibrosing colonopathy	0	Hepatitis – D and E	2
Food allergy	0	Hepatitis – neonatal	1
Foreign body ingestion	1	Hepatitis – viral complications	1
Free radical damage	0	Hepatobiliary dysfunction	3
Gag reflex	0	Hepatocellular carcinoma	1
Gallbladder	1	Hepatosplenomegaly	1
Gallstones	1	Hepatotoxicity	1
Gardener's syndrome	1	Hereditary spherocytosis	1
Gastrectomy	1	Hernia	3
Gastric ATPase pump (adult)	2	Hirschsprung's disease	2
Gastric emptying	0	HUS (haemolytic uraemic	
Gastric lymphoma	1	syndrome)	5
Gastric secretion	0	HUS – *Escherichia coli* O157	3
Gastrin	0	Hydrolysed protein formula	2
Gastritis	0	Hyperbilirubinaemia	2
Gastroenteritis (adult)	2	Hypercarotenosis	1
Gastroenteritis – acute	1	Hypoallergenic feeds	2
Gastrointestinal bleed (adult)	3	Inflammatory bowel disease	1
Gastro-oesophageal junction	0	Inflammatory bowel disease –	
Gastro-oesophageal reflux	4	Crohn's disease (adult)	11
Gastro-oesophageal reflux –		Inflammatory bowel disease –	
radiology	1	ulcerative colitis (adult)	8
Gastroschisis	1	Inflammatory liver disease	0
Giardia lamblia (adult)	6	Inspissated bile syndrome	1
Granuloma (adult)	1	Intestinal lymphangectasia	3
Gut radiology	1	Intestinal obstruction	1
Haematocolpos	1	Intussusception	3
Haematology	1	Irritable bowel syndrome	2
Haemochromatosis (adult)	3	Jaundice	4
Haemochromatosis – neonatal	1	Jaundice – conjugated (adult)	6

questions

questions

Teeth	0	Vitamin B3	0
Teeth – development	0	Vitamin B6	1
Tender scrotal swelling	1	Vitamin C	1
Tongue	1	Vitamin D (adult)	6
Total parenteral nutrition	0	Vitamin D – deficiency	1
Trace elements	0	Vitamin E	1
Tracheo-oesophageal atresia	2	Vitamin K	4
Tumours	1	Vitamin treatments	0
Turcot's syndrome	0	Vitamins	0
Ulceration	1	Volvulus	1
Umbilicus	1	Vomiting	5
Villous atrophy (adult)	2	Whipple's disease	1
Vitamin A	1	Xylose tolerance test	1
Vitamin B1	1	*Yersinia*	1
Vitamin B2	0	Zollinger–Ellison syndrome	1

Multiple True/False Questions

60 Which of the following statements regarding bloody diarrhoea is correct?

- ○ A should be treated with loperamide
- ○ B is due to bacterial infection in all cases
- ○ C is notifiable and requires the use of antibiotics
- ○ D can be associated with extraintestinal complications
- ○ E is always associated with an arthropathy

61 Anal fissures

- ○ A occur only in children
- ○ B will respond to sphincterotomy in the majority of cases
- ○ C produce a malaena stool
- ○ D are associated with child sexual abuse in all cases
- ○ E will heal at a faster rate with topical diazepam

62 With regard to appendicitis which of the following statements is true?

- ○ A It is associated with a 5% mortality rate in children in the UK
- ○ B The commonest complication in 0.05% of cases is wound infection
- ○ C Perforation leads to infertility in females
- ○ D It is associated with obstruction of the appendiceal lumen with faecolith(s)
- ○ E Spontaneous resolution does not occur

63 Regarding constipation, which of the following statements is true?

- ○ A It requires treatment with cisapride
- ○ B Treatment with lactulose is associated with flatulence and abdominal pain
- ○ C It is associated with an organic cause in 25% of cases
- ○ D In under-5-year-olds is associated with 50% recovery within 5 years
- ○ E In under-5-year-olds is associated with 65% recovery within 10 years

64 Which of the following statements regarding *Helicobacter pylori* colonisation are correct?

- ○ A This is causally related to the development of duodenal ulceration
- ○ B Eradication heals 83% of gastric ulcers within 6 weeks
- ○ C Eradication reduces dyspeptic symptoms
- ○ D Treatment for 2 weeks is better than 1 week of treatment in terms of eradicating the organism
- ○ E Eradication improves gastro-oesophageal reflux symptoms

questions

65 For children with mild-to-moderate dehydration associated with acute gastroenteritis, the intravenous route is superior in terms of which of the following:

- A Decreasing the duration of diarrhoea
- B Decreasing the time spent in hospital
- C Associated weight gain at the time of discharge
- D Increased complications
- E Giving better control of the blood electrolyte balance

66 Regarding gastro-oesophageal reflux which of the following statements are correct?

- A The associated clinical or endoscopic features of oesophagitis are improved by cimetidine over a 3-month period
- B Episodes of regurgitation are improved by the use of sodium alginate over 2 months
- C Treatment with cisapride is no longer recommended
- D The condition spontaneously resolves by 12–18 months in most normal children
- E It can be associated with haematemesis

67 Regarding infantile colic, which of the following statements is true?

- A It is due to child abuse in 35% of cases
- B It starts at 3 months of age and ceases by 1 year of life
- C It is caused by urinary tract infection
- D It is higher in bottle-fed babies than breast-fed babies
- E It is relieved by carrying the child for at least 4½ hours a day

68 Regarding breastfeeding, which of the following statements are true?

- A It should be stopped in breast-milk-jaundiced babies
- B It should be stopped in the developed world in human immunodeficiency virus-positive mothers
- C It can transfer significant amounts of immunoglobulins
- D It continues in the majority of children to school age
- E It provides 50% of the required calories by virtue of its lipid

69 Swallowing disorders may be due to which of the following?

- A Cleft palate disorders
- B A vascular ring
- C Achalasia
- D Choanal atresia
- E Myasthenia gravis

70 Which of the following regarding coeliac disease is true?

○ A Has a prevalence of up to 1% in Europe
○ B Is associated with rice and maize ingestion
○ C Is due to α-gliadin breakdown products
○ D Involves class II major histocompatibility complex molecules presenting short peptide antigens to CD4+ lymphocytes
○ E Is associated with villous hypertrophy

71 Inflammatory bowel disease is seen in association with which of the following?

○ A Anterior uveitis
○ B Sclerosing cholangitis
○ C Erythema nodosum
○ D Acanthosis nigrans
○ E Café-au-lait patches

72 A 7-month-old boy has been having large vomits since about 1 month of age. Which feature would not fit with the diagnosis of gastro-oesophageal reflux?

○ A Torticollis
○ B Recurrent chest infections
○ C Growth on the 90th centile for weight
○ D Haematemesis
○ E Neurological impairment

73 A 3-month-old child has had diarrhoea for the past 2 days with a 10% body weight loss during this period. Which of the following signs may be seen?

○ A Depressed fontanelle
○ B Loss of skin tone and elasticity
○ C Tachycardia
○ D Sunken eyes
○ E Moist mucous membranes

74 A 5-week-old girl may present with obstructive jaundice due to all of the following causes except one. Which is the incorrect cause?

○ A Choledochal cyst
○ B α_1-Anti-trypsin deficiency
○ C Extrahepatic biliary atresia
○ D Alagille's syndrome
○ E Gilbert's syndrome

questions

75 **All the following statements about medium-chain triglycerides are correct apart from which one?**

- ○ A Biliary salts aid their gut absorption
- Ø B They undergo hydrolysis by lipase
- ○ C They are metabolised in the liver cells
- ○ D They are carried on albumin
- ○ E They are taken up by chylomicrons to only to a small extent

Best of Five Questions

76 **A 6-month-old African child presents during the weaning phase, wasted with severe loss of weight to less than 60% of the international standard. He has profuse watery diarrhoea, and on examination he has over 10% dehydration, reduced subcutaneous fat and tissue but normal head growth. This child is diagnosed as having a form of protein–calorie malnutrition.**

What is the diagnosis for this child?

- ○ A Kwashiorkor
- ○ B Coeliac disease
- ○ C Marasmus
- ○ D Nutritional dwarfism
- ○ E Underweight

77 **A 4-year-old boy presents from a rural African country having suffered from malaria. On examination, you find a very slim child with marked muscle wasting, a positive flag sign (red hair), hepatomegaly and hypothermia. His skin has a flaky paint appearance, and his hair is wiry and red. He appears grossly oedematous, and his weight has fallen to less than 60–80% of the international standard. Examinations confirm decreased immunity with low IgE, low albumin and aminoaciduria. Thyroid function tests are abnormal.**

What is the diagnosis in the above clinical situation?

- ○ A Kwashiorkor
- ○ B Coeliac disease
- ○ C Marasmus
- ○ D Nutritional dwarfism
- ○ E Underweight

78 **You are handed a radiograph including a wrist that shows the following features:**

- **an irregular, splayed metaphysis**
- **generalised osteopenia**
- **a widened zone of provisional calcification at the sites of fastest growth (knee and wrist)**
- **metaphyseal cupping and splaying**
- **widening of the anterior costochondral junctions of the ribs**

What is the diagnosis?

○ A Osteomyelitis
○ B Skeletal dysplasia
○ C Thanatophoric dwarfism
○ D Rickets
○ E Vitamin D deficiency

Extended Matching Questions

79 Theme: Calcium Metabolism

A Acute pancreatitis
B X-linked hypophosphataemic rickets
C Both acute pancreatitis and X-linked hypophosphataemic rickets
D Neither acute pancreatitis nor X-linked hypophosphataemic rickets

From the above list, choose the item which is best associated with each of the statements below.

○ 1 Hypocalcaemia is a frequently seen feature
○ 2 This can be caused by sarcoidosis
○ 3 This condition may be treated using antibiotics
○ 4 This can be induced by alcohol

Genetics and Syndromes

Question Frequency

Genetics

Abnormal karyotype (adult)	2
Allele	0
Allelic expansion	0
Alphafetoprotein	2
Amniocentesis	2
Antenatal detection	1
Associations (adult)	1
Asthma	1
Autosomal co-dominance	2
Autosomal dominant (adult)	6
Autosomal recessive (adult)	6
Blindness	0
Chromosomal anomalies	3
Chromosomal breakages	2
Chromosomal inactivation	3
Chromosomal locations	1
Chromosome microdeletion	2
Clotting and genetics	0
Cystic fibrosis	3
Definitions	1
Fetal abnormalities	4
Fetal detection of diseases	2
Genders	0
Gene expression	0
Genes and malignancies	0
Genetic anticipation	5
Genetics of liver	0
Genomic imprinting	3

Hereditary cancers	0
High arched palate	0
Mendelian genetics	0
Mental retardation	2
Monozygotic twins	0
Mutation rates	0
Neonatal presentation	0
Patterns of inheritance	3
Single-gene disorders	0
Tissue sources for DNA analysis	0
Trinucleotide repeats	1
XL dominant	5
XL recessive (adult)	8

Syndromes

Achondroplasia	1
Aicardi's syndrome	1
Alagille's syndrome	1
Angelman's syndrome	2
Associations	0
Bardet–Biedl syndrome	0
Batten disease	1
Beckwith–Wiedemann syndrome	2
Bloom's syndrome	2
CAP syndrome	1
Cartilage–hair syndrome	1
Charcot–Marie–Tooth disease	0
CHARGE association	1
Cleft lip and palate	1

questions

Cleidocranial dysostosis	0	Osteogenesis imperfecta	1
Clinodactyly (adult)	2	Patau's syndrome	2
Cockayne's syndrome	1	Pendred's syndrome	2
Coloboma	1	Phocomelia	1
Conradi syndrome	1	Pierre Robin sequence	1
Cornelia de Lange's syndrome	1	Poland's syndrome	1
Cri du chat syndrome	1	Polydactyly	1
Down's syndrome	8	Prader–Willi syndrome syndrome	5
Drash syndrome	1	Pseudoxanthoma elasticum	0
Drug metabolism disorders	0	Rett's syndrome	1
Dwarfism	1	Riley–Day syndrome	1
Edward's syndrome	2	Rubenstein–Tabyi syndrome	2
Ehlers–Danlos syndrome	1	Russell–Silver syndrome	1
Ellis–van Creveld syndrome	1	Russell's diencephalic syndrome	1
Fetal alcohol syndrome (adult)	3	Schwachman–Diamond	
Fragile X syndrome (adult)	8	syndrome	1
Goldenhar's syndrome	1	Seckel's syndrome	1
Hereditery telangiectasia	1	Septo-optic dysplasia	1
Holt–Oram syndrome	1	Smith–Lemli–Opitz syndrome	2
Hypertrichosis	1	Soto's syndrome	1
Killian–Pallo syndrome	0	Spondyloepiphyseal dysplasia	1
Klinefelter's syndrome (adult)	6	Stickler's syndrome	1
Klippel–Feil syndrome syndrome	1	Submentality	0
Laurence–Moon–Biedl syndrome	2	Supravalvular aortic stenosis	3
LEOPARD syndrome	1	Syndactyly	1
Linkage associations	0	TAR syndrome	1
Lowe's syndrome	0	Thanatophoric dwarfism	1
Macroglossia	0	TORCH syndrome	1
Mandibular hypoplasia	1	Treacher Collins syndrome	2
Marcus Gunn's syndrome	1	Turner's syndrome	6
Meckel–Gruber syndrome	1	Usher's syndrome	1
Micrognathia	1	VATER association	1
Neck mobility	1	Waardenburg's syndrome	1
Noonan's syndrome (adult)	6	WAGR syndrome	1
Nuchal thickening	0	Williams' syndrome	3
Oculofacial digital syndrome	1	XYY adult	2

Multiple True/False Questions

80 A child with Down's syndrome may have which of the following phenotypic features?

- A Brachycephaly
- B Tall stature
- C Hypertonia in the neonatal period
- D Fifth finger clinodacytyly
- E Duodenal atresia

81 Which of the following are true for Alagille's syndrome?

- A It is only autosomal dominantly inheritable
- B It clinically portrays posterior embryotoxin
- C It is not complicated by chronic cholestasis
- D It requires investigations such as spinal radiography and splenic biopsy
- E Its differential diagnosis includes Zellweger's syndrome

82 Which of the following are the major criteria for the diagnosis of tuberous sclerosis?

- A Bone cysts
- B Multiple renal cysts
- C Gingival fibroma
- D Non-renal hamartoma
- E Hamartomatous rectal polyps

83 Which of the following cause in-curving of the fifth finger?

- A Seckel's syndrome
- B Rubinstein-Taybi's syndrome
- C Carpenter's syndrome
- D Cornelia de Lange's syndrome
- E All of the above

84 What form of inheritance does Chédiak–Higashi syndrome have?

- A Autosomal dominant
- B Autosomal recessive
- C Co-dominance
- D X-linked recessive
- E X-linked dominant

Best of Five Questions

85 You review an 8-year-old boy who attends a school for moderate learning difficulties. His neonatal history includes intrauterine growth retardation, neonatal hypotonia and hypoglycaemia. He was a difficult feeder and required nasogastric feeds. As an infant, he became obese. On entry to nursery school, he was referred for eating soil, paper and other objects. On examination, the boy has short stature, mild dysmorphism with almond-shaped eyes and a downturned fish-mouth appearance. He has small hands and feet, and hypogonadism. He has speech and language delay with poor development progression.

What is the most likely diagnosis?

- A Disorder of paternal uniparental disomy
- B Disorder of maternal uniparental disomy
- C Angelman's syndrome
- D Beckwith–Wiedemann syndrome
- E Turner's syndrome

86 You review a child at a school for severe learning difficulties. Her previous medical history includes microcephaly and global developmental delay, and she is being treated with vigabatrin for infantile spasms. On examination, you encounter a fair-haired, blue-eyed girl with coarse facies and prognathism who appears to be very happy and claps her hands as she enters the room. She is hypotonic with an ataxic gait. Neuromuscular examination reveals a left-sided scoliosis. She has a characteristic EEG abnormality.

What is the possible diagnosis for this girl?

- A Trisomy 15
- B Disorder of genomic imprinting
- C Paternal uniparental disomy for chromosome 15
- D Maternal uniparental disomy for chromosome 15
- E Presence of the 15q gene

87 You review a 7-year-old boy with possible medulloblastoma. His antenatal history includes microcephaly, intrauterine growth retardation and hypoglycaemia. The postnatal period was complicated by recurrent infections, including serous otitis media, urinary tract infections and tonsillitis. The child initially presented to a child development centre with ataxia, hypotonia, short stature and global developmental delay. On examination, you find a small child who looks mildly dysmorphic and is wearing a sun hat. He has fair hair, blue eyes and multiple freckles.

What is the possible diagnosis here?

○ A Louis–Bar's syndrome
○ B Ataxia telangiectasia
○ C Bloom's syndrome
○ D Xeroderma pigmentosum
○ E Incontinentia pigmenti

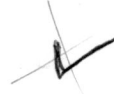

88 An 8-month-old girl presents with a history of atrial septal defect and duplex kidneys and has had a successful repair of her cleft lip and palate. A cranial ultrasound scan shows multiple choroid plexus cysts. On examination, you find a small child with micrognathia, low-set ears and a prominent forehead and occiput. She has hypoplastic nails with an overlapping index and middle finger. Her rocker-bottom feet show no evidence of lymphoedema. Cardiovascular examination reveals a short sternum with a 2/6 pansystolic murmur at the upper left sternal edge radiating to the apex.

Which of the following diagnoses is possible in this case?

○ A Pierre Robin sequence
○ B Velocardiofacial syndrome
○ C Patau's syndrome
○ D Edward's syndrome
○ E Treacher Collins syndrome

89 You review a 48-hour-old male infant whose mother suffered from memory loss and hypoglycaemia during pregnancy. The amniocentesis result is normal. You find a child with intrauterine growth retardation, all growth measurements being less than the 0.4th centile. The child is irritable and has feeding difficulties. On examination, the child is microcephalic, with microphthalmia, hypertelorism and retrognathia. He has short palpable fissures, a small philtrum with a thin upper lip and maxillary hypoplasia. Cardiovascular examination reveals a 2/6 ejection systolic murmur at the lower left sternal edge, radiating to the apex. A differential diagnosis for cardiac abnormalities and maxillary hypoplasia is given below.

What is the probable diagnosis in this case?

- A Marfan's syndrome
- B Maternal phenylketonuria
- C Rubinstein–Taybi's syndrome
- D Fetal alcohol syndrome
- E Turner's syndrome

90 You are called to resuscitate and ventilate a 32+6 week gestation infant who is found to have breathing difficulties. Oligohydramnios and small kidneys were noted antenatally. On examination, the baby shows growth retardation. The main problems include difficulty in ventilation, requiring high pressures and oxygenation, a poor urine output and hypoglycaemia. On investigation, the child has hypoplastic lungs and bilateral renal agenesis.

What is the diagnosis?

- A Infant of an insulin-dependent diabetes mellitus mother
- B Hepatitis A
- C Infectious mononucleosis
- D Potter's syndrome
- E Maternal antiretroviral disease

91 The diagnostic criteria for neurofibromatosis type I are fulfilled by one of the following

- A There are two or more café-au-lait spots
- B There is axillary freckling
- C There is groin freckling and a plexiform neurofibroma
- D There is one neurofibroma and two café-au-lait spots
- E There are six café-au-lait spots and groin freckling

92 You review a boy with a blood sugar level of 2.1 mmol/l. The previous medical history includes macrosomia, neonatal hypoglycaemia, hypocalcaemia and polycythaemia, and he has been successfully treated for an omphalocele. On examination, he is a large infant with exophthalmos and hemihypertrophy. On abdominal palpation, there is a ballotable left mass. The child has a large tongue and a distinctive earlobe abnormality. Investigations show hyperinsulinaemia with associated hypokalaemia and hypomagnesaemia.

1   *What might the visceromegaly be due to?*

○ A Wilms' tumour with hemihypertrophy
○ B Adrenal cortical adenoma
○ C Hepatoblastoma
○ D Neuroblastoma
○ E Medulloblastoma

2   *What is the likely diagnosis?*

○ A Soto's syndrome
○ B Cerebral gigantism
○ C Beckwith–Wiedemann's syndrome
○ D Bloom's syndrome
○ E Laurence–Moon–Biedl syndrome

Extended Matching Questions

93 Theme: Karyotype abnormalities

    A Burkitt's lymphoma
    B Chronic granulocytic leukaemia
    C Cri du chat syndrome
    D Pierre Robin sequence
    E Huntington's chorea
    F Klinefelter's syndrome
    G Meningomyelocele
    H Edwards' syndrome
    I Patau's syndrome
    J Phenylketonuria

Which of the above diseases is/are associated with each of the karyotype abnormalities mentioned below?

○ 1 Reciprocal translocation of part of the long arm of chromosome 22 to chromosome 9
○ 2 Abnormality on the c8 locus of chromosome 4

○ 3 Trisomy 13
○ 4 Trisomy 18
○ 5 A karyotype that cannot be established
○ 6 Translocation 8:14

94 Theme: Forms of inheritance

A Hereditary spherocytosis
B Holt–Oram syndrome
C Congenital adrenal hyperplasia
D α1-Antitrypsin deficiency
E Neurofibromatosis types I and II
F Friedreich's ataxia
G Sickle cell anaemia
H β-Thalassaemia
I Noonan's syndrome
J Xeroderma pigmentosum

Match the above disorders to the relevant form of inheritance.

○ 1 Which of the above show *autosomal dominance* inheritance?
○ 2 Which of the above show *autosomal recessive* inheritance?
○ 3 Which of the above show *co-dominant* inheritance?

95 Theme: Anticipation

A Marfan's disease
B Fragile X syndrome (type A)
C Friedreich's ataxia
D Spinocerebellar atrophy type I
E Myotonic dystrophy
F Huntington's chorea
G Spinomuscular atrophy
H Cystic fibrosis
I Homocystinuria
J Kartagener's syndrome

The diseases above show anticipation. Match the relevant diseases to one of the following categories:

○ 1 Untranslated trinucleotide repeats
○ 2 Translated trinucleotide repeats
○ 3 Negative trinucleotide repeats

96 Theme: Pedigree maps

A Autosomal dominant inheritance
B Autosomal recessive inheritance
C X-linked dominant inheritance

D X-linked recessive inheritance
E Maternal mitochondrially inherited diseases

Match the following three pedigree maps to one of the forms of inheritance above.

○ 1 Pedigree map 1

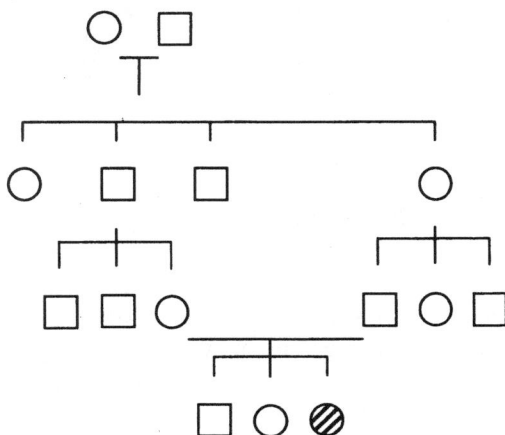

○ 2 Pedigree map 2

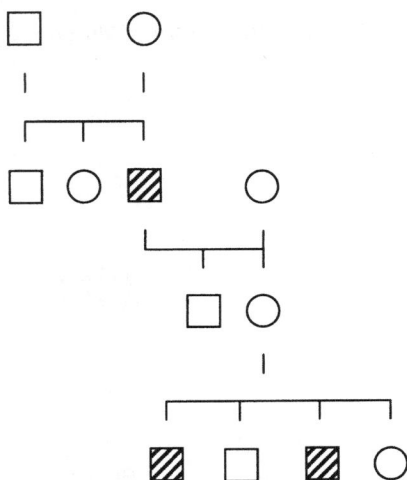

○ 3 Pedigree map 3

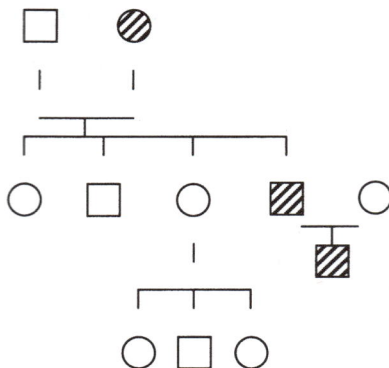

97 Theme: X-linked inheritance

- A Ichthyosis
- B Retinitis pigmentosa
- C Vitamin D-resistant rickets
- D Severe combined immune deficiency
- E Goltz syndrome
- F Incontinentia pigmenti
- G Orofacial digital syndrome
- H Alport's syndrome
- I Fragile X syndrome
- J Lesch–Nyhan syndrome

The above ten diseases show X-linked inheritance. Match the diseases above to their form of inheritance.

1 X-linked dominant inheritance.
2 X-linked recessive inheritance.
3 Both of the above.

98 Theme: Genetic pedigree

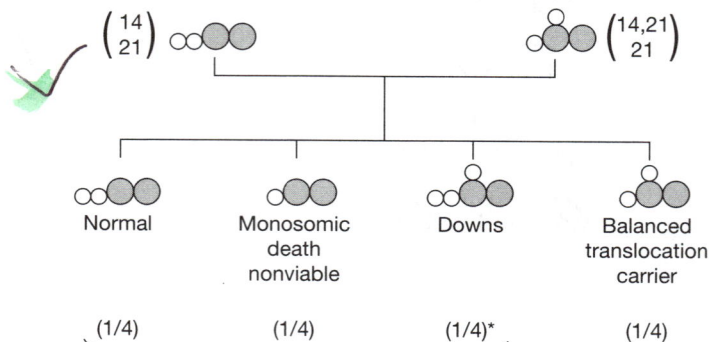

A 1%
B 2%
C 3%
D 4%
E 5%
F 6%
G 7%
H 8%
I 9%
J 10%

Match the results above to the three questions below.

○ 1 What is the carrier rate for the mother?
○ 2 What is the carrier rate for the father?
○ 3 What is the percentage of mosaicism?

99 Theme: Genetic Syndromes

A Noonan's syndrome
B Laurence–Moon–Biedl syndrome
C Patau's syndrome
D Fragile X syndrome
E Rubinstein–Taybi's syndrome
F Smith–Lemli–Opitz syndrome
G Turner's syndrome
H Williams' syndrome
I Down's syndrome
J Prader–Willi syndrome

Match the three clinical scenarios to one of the ten diagnoses above.

○ 1 A child presents for follow-up blood tests. Previous medical problems include failure to thrive, microcephaly, learning difficulties and nephrocalcinosis secondary to hypertension. The previous medical history includes hypercalcaemia, hypercalciuria and secondary hypercalcinosis. On examination, this child has elfin-like facies with hyperacusis and a hoarse voice. He has a stellate iris. Cardiovascular examination depicts aortic stenosis. What is the diagnosis?

○ 2 A child presents with a genetic disorder. Previous medical problems include microcephaly, moderate learning difficulties, hypotonia and autistic features. On examination, the child appears to have a prominent jaw line, a long face and large ears, with a high-arched palate. He has macro-orchidism and is post-pubertal. He is found to have hypotonia and hyperextensible and lax joints. What is the underlying diagnosis?

questions

○ 3 A child presents with seizures, microcephaly, aortic stenosis, cryptorchidism and duplex kidneys. He is known to have cholesterol reductase deficiency. On examination, he has a prominent forehead, low-set ears and bilateral ptosis. Cardiovascular examination reveals a 2/6 ejection systolic murmur at the right second intercostal space radiating to the carotids. The child has a clenched left hand and syndactyly of the second and third toes. He is intermittently hypotonic with increased reflexes bilaterally. A high-cholesterol diet has improved his personality but not his learning difficulty. What is his likely diagnosis is?

100 Theme: Genetic Syndromes

    A Noonan's syndrome
    B Laurence–Moon–Biedl syndrome
    C Patau's syndrome
    D Fragile X syndrome
    E Rubinstein–Taybi's syndrome
    F Smith–Lemli–Opitz syndrome
    G Turner's syndrome
    H Williams' syndrome
    I Down's syndrome
    J Prader–Willi syndrome

Match the three clinical scenarios to one of the ten above diagnoses.

○ 1 A child presents with short stature, deafness, cryptorchidism and pulmonary stenosis. On examination, he is found to have hypertelorism, an antimongoloid slant of the eyes, low-set ears, micrognathia and a high-arched palate. Cardiovascular examination reveals a 3/6 ejection systolic murmur at the upper left sternal second intercostal space. He has marked webbing of the neck, pectus carinatum and pectus excavatum. The musculoskeletal system displays a cubitus valgus but no other abnormality. What is a possible diagnosis?

○ 2 You review a 4-day-old female infant on the special care baby unit with intrauterine growth retardation and feeding difficulties. On examination, the child is found to have microcephaly, cutis aplasia and jaundice. There are mild dysmorphic features, including low-set ears, micrognathia, a small nose and a submucous cleft palate. Posterior axial polydactyly of the hands and feet is obvious. On examination, the child has a 3/6 ejection systolic murmur at the lower left sternal edge radiating to the apex. A cranial ultrasound scan confirms holoprosencephaly. What is the diagnosis?

○ 3 In a genetics clinic, you observe an obese boy with short stature who clearly has learning difficulties. His previous medical problems include short stature, hypothalamic hyperplasia, cranial diabetes insipidus and hypogonadism. He is being reviewed by the ophthalmologists for night blindness and retinitis pigmentosa. What is his possible diagnosis?

Haematology

Question Frequency

ABO and rhesus incompatibility	1	Blood film (adult)	2
Anaemia – bone pain	0	Blood products	0
Anaemia – chronic disease (adult)	6	Bone marrow (adult)	2
Anaemia – cold autoimmune	3	Bone marrow transplantation	0
Anaemia – Fanconi's (adult)	5	Clotting – factor V leiden	1
Anaemia – haemolytic (adult)	8	Clotting cascade	3
Anaemia – hypochromia (adult)	7	Coagulation tests	3
Anaemia – hypochromic		Coombs test (adult)	2
microcytic	5	Cryoglobulinaemia	2
Anaemia – hypoplastic	3	Cryoprecipitate	0
Anaemia – iron deficiency (adult)	5	Diamond–Blackfan syndrome	2
Anaemia – leukoerythroblastic	1	Disseminated intravascular	
Anaemia – megaloblastic (adult)	7	coagulation (adult)	1
Anaemia – normochromic		Eosinophils (adult)	4
normocytic	3	Epidemiology	0
Anaemia – sideroblastic (adult)	6	Erythrocytes	0
APCR	2	Erythrocytosis (adult)	1
Aplasia – dyskeratosis	1	Erythropoiesis (adult)	1
Aplasia – red cell	1	Erythropoietin	0
Aplastic anaemia (adult)	8	Factor VIII deficiency	3
Aspirin	0	Factor XIII deficiency	2
Associations (adult)	1	Fanconi syndrome	3
Atypical mononuclear cells (adult)	2	Filaria	0
Basal naevus syndrome	0	Foam cell	1
Basophilia (adult)	2	Folic acid (adult)	5
Bernard–Soulier syndrome	1	Fresh frozen plasma	5
Bleeding tendency (adult)	7	G-CSF	0
Bleeding time (adult)	7	Glanzmann's thrombasthenia	1

questions

Glucose-6-phosphate-dehydrogenase deficiency	7	Myelodysplastic syndrome	0
Haemoglobin	3	Myeloid line white cells	0
Haemoglobin – glycosylated	0	Myelosclerosis (adult)	1
Haemoglobinopathies	1	Neutropenia (adult)	2
Haemolysis	1	Neutropenia – cyclical	1
Haemophagocytic histiocytosis	1	Neutrophils	0
Haemophilia (adult)	4	Pancytopenia (adult)	6
Haemopoietin	0	Paroxymal nocturnal haemoglobinuria	1
Hepatosplenomegaly	1	Plasma volumes	1
Hereditary bleeding disorders	1	Platelets	0
Hereditary Haem telangiectasia	0	Polycythaemia (adult)	2
Hereditary spherocytosis (adult)	7	Polycythaemia – rubra vera (adult)	2
Hodgkin's disease (adult)	5	Purpura	0
Hyposplenism/hypersplenism	4	Pyruvate kinase deficiency	1
Idiopathic thrombocytopenic (adult) purpura	8	Reticulocytes	4
Iron overload	4	Schilling test	1
Iron therapy	8	Sezary syndrome	0
Kleihauer stain	1	Shwachman's syndrome	3
Langerhans cell hystiocytosis	3	Sickle cell disease (adult)	7
Leukaemia – acute lymphoblastic (adult)	4	Sickle cell disease – haemoglobin C disease	1
Leukaemia – acute myeloid (adult)	6	Sickle cell disease – hyposthenurea	1
Leukaemia – chronic lymphoblastic (adult)	4	Splenectomy (adult)	5
		Splenomegaly (adult)	5
Leukaemia – chronic myeloid (adult)	3	Thalassaemia – alpha major	5
Leukaemia – hairy cell (adult)	3	Thalassaemia – beta trait	5
Leukaemia – lymphoid (adult)	4	Thalassaemia – genetics	3
Leukoerythroblastic blood picture	1	Thalassaemia – major	5
Lipoma	1	Thrombocytopenia (adult)	4
Lymphadenopathy (adult)	1	Thrombocytopenia – chronic idiopathic (adult)	4
Lymphocytosis	0	Thrombocytosis (adult)	2
Macrocytosis (adult)	4	Transfusion reactions	1
Marrow hypoplasia	2	Venous thromboembolism	0
Mast cells	0	Vitamin B12 (adult)	5
Methaemoglobinaemia (adult)	6	Von Hippel–Lindau disease	0
Microcytosis	1	Von Willebrand's disease	7
Monocytosis	1	Wiscott–Aldrich sydrome	3
Mycosis fungoides (adult)	1	Xenotransplantation	1

Multiple True/False Questions

101 Causes of platelet dysfunction include which of the following?

- ○ A Alcohol
- ○ B Uraemia
- ○ C Acute myeloid leukaemia
- ○ D Penicillin
- ○ E Disseminated intravascular coagulation

102 Causes of red blood cell fragmentation include which of the following?

- ○ A March haemoglobinuria
- ○ B Hepatic disease
- ○ C Renal disease
- ○ D Diabetes insipidus
- ○ E Haemolytic–uraemic syndrome (HUS)

103 β-Thalassaemia major is associated with which of the following?

- ○ A A decreased level of HbA_2
- ○ B A decreased level of HbF
- ○ C A decreased level of erythropoietin
- ○ D An increased frequency of fractures
- ○ E Hepatosplenomegaly

Best of Five Questions

104 A 2½-year-old Italian boy presents with a 12-hour history of nausea, vomiting and anorexia after he had ingested cola and beans for dinner. He is on a course of penicillin for a throat infection. On examination, you find that he is slightly jaundiced, with cervical lymphadenopathy and hepatomegaly. Investigations show a leukocytosis with acute non-spherocytic haemolysis on the blood film.

One possible diagnosis is

- ○ A Paroxysmal nocturnal haemoglobinuria
- ○ B Hereditary spherocytosis
- ○ C Aplastic anaemia secondary to parvovirus infection
- ○ D A haemoglobinopathy
- ○ E Glucose-6-phosphate dehydrogenase deficiency

105 With the above disorder in mind, a genetic test is sent off and family studies commenced. What form of inheritance may this disorder show?

- A Autosomal dominant
- B Autosomal recessive
- C X-linked dominant
- D X-linked recessive
- E Co-dominant

106 A 3-year-old girl presents with a 7-day history of an upper respiratory tract infection. She has suffered a prodromal coryzal illness with epistaxis for 3 weeks. On examination, she is pale, and has multiple purpura and bruises with mucosal bleeding. Cardiovascular, respiratory and abdominal examination is unremarkable. A full blood count confirms thrombocytopenia. A blood film shows that the girl has an autoimmune haemolytic anaemia with normal blood elements. A bone marrow biopsy confirms an increase in megakaryocytes and platelet turnover. The likely diagnosis is:

- A Acute myeloid leukaemia
- B Evans' syndrome
- C Acute lymphocytic leukaemia
- D Drug-induced autoimmune haemolytic anaemia
- E Meningococcal septicaemia

107 A 4-year-old north European boy presents with anaemia and jaundice. His previous medical history includes neonatal jaundice, and he has recently suffered a viral upper respiratory tract infection. On examination, he is small and pale with a slapped-cheek appearance and jaundiced sclera. Cardiovascular and respiratory examination is unremarkable. On palpation of the abdomen, splenomegaly is noted. Investigations confirm pancytopenia, hypochromic anaemia, a negative Coombs test, a decreased red cell concentration and a low reticulocyte count. A blood film shows an abnormality. There is increased haemolysis on the osmotic fragility test, and the boy has a raised zinc and a reduced folate level.

1   *What is the organism most likely to have caused his upper respiratory tract illness?*

○   A   Herpes simplex virus
○   B   Parainfluenza B virus
○   C   Parvovirus B19
○   D   Adenovirus
○   E   Respiratory syncytial virus

2   *With the above infection in mind, what is a possible diagnosis for the pancytopenia?*

○   A   Zinc poisoning
○   B   Iron deficiency anaemia
○   C   β-Thalassaemia major
○   D   Hereditary spherocytosis
○   E   ABO incompatibility

3   *What major abnormality was found on the blood film?*

○   A   Many reticulocyte cells
○   B   Sickle cells
○   C   Helmet cells
○   D   Spheroidal cells
○   E   Howell–Jolly bodies

4   *With the above diagnosis in mind, what is the likely form of inheritance?*

○   A   Autosomal dominant
○   B   Autosomal recessive
○   C   X-linked dominant
○   D   X-linked recessive
○   E   Co-dominant

Extended Matching Questions

108 Theme: Resuscitation fluids

    A   Hypoalbuminaemic oedema
    B   Nephritic syndrome
    C   Disseminated intravascular coagulation
    D   Thrombotic thrombocytopenic purpura
    E   Nephrotic syndrome
    F   Major burns
    G   Persistent bleeding (high prothrombin time)
    H   Liver disease
    I   Surgery to the biliary tract
    J   Factor II, V, VII and IX deficiency

Of the ten clinical scenarios above:

○○○○ 1 Which **four** may be treated with fresh frozen plasma?
○○○○ 2 Which **four** may be treated with 5% human albumin?
　　○ 3 Which **one** may be treated with clotting factors?

109 Theme: Clotting profiles

A Full blood count – normal
B Clotting profile – increased activated partial thromboplastin time (APTT)
C Film – normal platelets
D Decreased factor VIII von Willebrand activation
E Decreased factor VIIIC activation
F Decreased factor VIII procoagulation activity
G Decreased factor VIII antigen activity
H Prolonged bleeding time
I Normal aggregation to ADP and collagen
J Decreased platelet activation to risocetin

A 4-year-old male presents with mucosal bleeding, epistaxis and bruises. The haematological results above were obtained.

○ 1 A differential diagnosis is given below. What is the diagnosis?

A Haemophilia A
B Haemophilia B
C Christmas disease
D Von Willebrand's disease
E Bernard–Soulier disease

○ 2 With the above diagnosis in mind, what is the form of inheritance?

A Autosomal dominant
B Autosomal recessive
C X-linked dominant
D X-linked recessive
E Co-dominant

110 Theme: Pancytopenia

A Aplastic anaemia
B Paroxysmal nocturnal haemoglobinuria
C Acute lymphoblastic leukaemia
D Acute myeloid leukaemia
E Gaucher's disease
F Haemosiderosis
G Drug-induced marrow aplasia
H Stage IV neuroblastoma
I Miliary tuberculosis
J Severe haemolytic–uraemic syndrome

Match the following three clinical scenarios to the above ten aetiological factors for pancytopenia.

○ 1 A 4-year-old boy presents to the A&E department with pallor and bruising. A full blood count shows pancytopenia. Which six of the above cause pancytopenia *without* splenomegaly?

○ 2 A 6-year-old girl presents to the A&E department with pallor and bruises with splenomegaly. Which four of the above disorders are consistent with pancytopenia and *associated* splenomegaly?

○ 3 A 10-year-old boy presents with pallor, bruising and hepatosplenomegaly. Which five of the above disorders are consistent with pancytopenia and *hepatosplenomegaly*?

111 Theme: Methaemoglobinaemia

A Paraquat
B Vitamin D
C Primaquine
D Nitrates
E Potassium chlorate
F Quinones
G Ascorbic acid
H Chloroquine
I Dapsone
J Methylene blue

An 8-year-old girl returns from a holiday in Africa to her farm in Gloucestershire with an acute onset of cyanosis and difficulty in breathing. She is diagnosed with methaemoglobinaemia. Consider the ten drugs above.

○ 1 Which five may have caused the onset of the methaemoglobinaemia?
○ 2 Which two would be helpful in treating the methaemoglobinaemia?
○ 3 Which two have no association with her illness?

HIV/AIDS

Question Frequency

questions

Multiple True/False Questions

112 Regarding the human immunodeficiency virus (HIV)

○ A Early diagnosis and treatment of sexually transmitted disease reduces the risk of HIV infection within a 2-year period

○ B If untreated, 50% of patients will die from AIDS within 10 years

○ C HIV can be transmitted transplacentally

○ D It is due to 14 different types of virus

○ E The virus can be taken up by mucosal cells

113 With human immunodeficiency virus (HIV)

○ A The use of a two-nucleoside analogue drug regime (double therapy), compared with a protease inhibitor with two nucleoside drug analogues (triple therapy), is associated with a 50% decrease in the risk of death over 1 year

○ B Triple therapy is likely to decrease the likelihood of resistance compared with double therapy

○ C Zidovudine and either another nucleoside analogue or a protease inhibitor, compared with using zidovudine alone, significantly reduces the risk of AIDS-defining illness in groups followed up between 1 and 3 years

○ D The risk of infection is at least 2–5 times greater in people with other sexually transmitted diseases

○ E Presumptive mass treatment for infection in people with other sexually transmitted diseases has decreased the incidence of retroviral infection in a 20-month study

114 In relation to mother-to-child transmission

○ A Zidovudine reduces the incidence of human immunodeficiency virus (HIV) in infants in studies with a follow-up of up to 18 months

○ B The duration of giving zidovudine has no effect on the rate of vertical transmission

○ C There is no difference between nevirapine and zidovudine in the rate of vertical transmission

○ D Giving multivitamins to pregnant women reduces the risk of fetal infection

○ E The risk of transmission is increased if there is a detectable viraemia

115 In human immunodeficiency virus (HIV) infection, aciclovir reduces opportunistic infection with which of the following?

○ A Herpes simplex virus
○ B Varicella zoster virus
○ C Cytomegalovirus
○ D *Toxoplasma gondii*
○ E *Candida albicans*

116 Co-trimoxazole reduces which of the following?

○ A Herpes simplex virus
○ B Varicella zoster virus
○ C *Toxoplasma gondii*
○ D *Candida albicans*
○ E *Pneumocystis carinii* pneumonia

Immunology

Question Frequency

Abcesses	1	Colony-stimulating factors	0
Acute-phase proteins	0	Complement	4
Adenosine deaminase deficiency	0	Cytokines	1
Adhesive glycoprotein deficiency	2	Fetal immunity and development	1
AI polyglandular adenopathy	1	Haemagglutinins	0
AIDS	1	Hereditary angio-oedema (adult)	7
Allergic rhinitis (adult)	1	HLA B27	0
Anaphylactic shock	0	Host pathogens	0
Antibodies	0	Human leukocyte antigens	3
Antigen-presenting cells	0	Hyper IgE syndrome	2
Antiglomerular basement		Hypersensitivity (adult)	5
membrane Aby	1	Hypersensitivity – type 1	0
Antinuclear antibodies	0	Hypersensitivity – type 3	4
Antinuclear cytoplasmic		Hypersensitivity – type 4	3
antibodies (ANCA)	0	Hypogammaglobulinaemia	3
Antiphospholipid antibody		IgA	2
syndrome	2	IgA deficiency	4
Arachidonic acid	0	IgD	2
Associations	1	IgE	2
Atopic dermatitis	0	IgG subclass deficiency	1
Autoimmune disorders	0	IgM	2
B-cell defects	0	Immune defects	2
Boils	1	Immune preparation	0
Cell-mediated immunity (adult)	1	Immune response	2
Cellular immunity	0	Immunocompromised host	0
Chediak–Higashi syndrome (adult)	2	Immunodeficiencies – primary	4
Chronic granulomatosis disease		Immunodeficiencies – severe	
(adult)	3	combined	0

questions

Multiple True/False Questions

117 Which of the following pathogens are associated with the accompanying immune disorder?

- A Mycobacteria and type 1 cytokine defects
- B Gram-negative bacteria and complement deficiency
- C Enterovirus and antibody defects
- D *Staphylococcus* and complement deficiency
- E *Meningococcus* and neutrophil defect

118 Which of the following statements regarding chronic cutaneous candidiasis are true?

- A It is associated with poor T-cell function
- B It can be successfully treated with bone marrow transplantation
- C It is totally eradicated with fluconazole
- D It can cause failure to gain weight in infancy
- E It may be associated with an endocrinopathy in adult life

119 Which of the following children should not receive live vaccines?

- A Those requiring regular intravenous immunoglobulin therapy
- B Those on a prednisolone dose of 3 mg/kg per day for longer than 1 week
- C Children with graft-versus-host disease
- D Children on chemotherapy
- E Children who have had a solid organ transplant

120 In which of the following diseases should a complement abnormality be suspected?

- A Recurrent folliculitis
- B *Pneumocystis carinii* infection
- C Recurrent swelling after trauma
- D Delayed separation of the cord
- E Pancreatitis

Best of Five Questions

121 This substance is derived from arachidonic acid. The arachidonic acid is cleaved into cyclooxygenase derivatives and lipoxygenase derivatives. This substance is produced by the latter and is synthesised by leukocytes and mast cells. Leukocytes and mast cells are mediators of inflammation and allergic reactions by increasing chemotaxis and vascular permeability and inducing smooth muscle constriction. They also cause arteriolar constriction and bronchoconstriction. What is the substance?

- A Thromboxane
- B Prostacyclin
- C Prostaglandin
- D Leukotriene
- E Eosinophil

122 An 18-month-old male presents with recurrent pneumonia, ear infections and tonsillitis. The family history includes a previous male infant death at 2 years of age from pneumococcal meningitis. The parents are therefore very concerned and wish further investigations to be carried out.

1   *Which of the following investigations would be most appropriate?*

- A T-cell function tests
- B Immunoglobulins and antibody responses to immunisation
- C OKT3 measurement
- D Phytohemagglutinin (PHA) test
- E Bone marrow aspiration

After the results have returned, it is found that the child has absent or decreased levels of immunoglobulins A, G and M. He has reduced responses to blood group antibodies to immunisations and an increased percentage of E rosettes with red blood cells. His PHA and nitroblue tetrazolium (NBT) tests are normal.

2   *The following differential diagnosis may be considered, but the ultimate disorder is which of the following?*

- A Common variable immune deficiency
- B X-linked agammaglobulinaemia
- C Chronic granulomatous disease
- D Severe combined immunodeficiency syndrome
- E Chédiak–Higashi syndrome

3   Which of the following are appropriate treatments for X-linked
     agammaglobulinaemia (more than one answer may be given)?

○ A A course of benzylpenicillin for an acute pneumonia and tonsillitis
○ B Azithromycin for 3 days every fortnight as a prophylactic antibiotic
○ C Intravenous immunoglobulin
○ D A booster vaccine to DPT, Hib and meningitis C
○ E Bone marrow transplantation

**123 A 4-year-old, fair-haired, fair-skinned child presents to the
outpatient department with a history of recurrent chest
infections, ataxia and muscle weakness. He has a long history
of fatigue and malaise, and a GP has wondered whether he
suffers from infectious mononucleosis. He is currently on
sodium valproate for seizures, which have been observed since
the age of 2 years. On examination, he has bilateral nystagmus,
photophobia and an increased red light reflex. He shows signs
of sensory and motor neuropathy, and marked muscle
weakness.**

1   Which of the following is the most likely informative investigation to be
     undertaken?

○ A Full blood count
○ B Clotting profile
○ C Bacterial and viral serology
○ D Chromosomal studies
○ E White cell count and natural killer cell function tests

2   What is the most probable diagnosis?

○ A Wilms' tumour
○ B Chédiak–Higashi syndrome
○ C Infectious mononucleosis
○ D Epstein–Barr virus-driven Burkitt's lymphoma
○ E Guillain–Barré syndrome

questions

124 A 4-month-old male infant is referred with a chronic history of superficial skin abscesses and painful lymphadenopathy. Routine investigations reveal chronic anaemia and neutrophilia with a raised erythrocyte sedimentation rate, and Gram-positive cocci have grown in a pus sample obtained from a peri-anal abscess 4 weeks previously. On examination, you find a pale child with a marked swelling of the left submandibular region. He has reduced air entry with crepitations at the left lower lobe consistent with a left lower lobe pneumonia. Abdominal examination reveals hepatomegaly and previous scarring from peri-anal abscesses. Routine sputum and stool samples are sent from the clinic, which reveal that he has grown *Serratia marcescens* from his sputum sample. He has had *Salmonella* infection in the previous 3 months.

1   Which is the most informative investigation to consider?

○ Ⓐ Immunoglobulin levels
○ B Skin biopsy of an abscess lesion
○ C Nitroblue tetrazolium (NBT) test
○ D Clotting screen
○ E Neutrophil function test

2   Appropriate management on discharge may be which of the following?

○ A Prophylactic antibiotics
○ B Amphotericin
○ C White cell and granulocyte infusions
○ D Interferon-λ infusions
○ Ⓔ All of the above

3   The diagnosis is which of the following?

○ A Chédiak–Higashi syndrome
○ Ⓑ Chronic granulomatous disease
○ C Lactoferrin deficiency
○ D Shwachman syndrome
○ E Systemic lupus erythematosus

4   What is the pattern of inheritance (there may be more than one answer)?

○ Ⓐ Autosomal dominance inheritance
○ Ⓑ Autosomal recessive inheritance
○ Ⓒ X-linked recessive inheritance
○ D X-linked dominant inheritance
○ E Co-dominant inheritance

125 A 15-year-old girl presents to the outpatient clinic with a chronic history of abdominal pain at the time of her menstrual cycle. Her parents have wondered whether she has been in contact with any environmental pollens or grasses, as at times she has a hoarse voice and her skin comes out in mild oedematous swellings. The parents feel that this could be a psychosomatic element, as it often occurs at times of illness, stress and cold. On examination, there is no fever, rash, arthropathy or oedema. Cardiovascular, respiratory and abdominal examination is unremarkable.

1   *A possible diagnosis could be which of the following?*

○ A Idiopathic chronic urticaria
○ B Systemic lupus erythematosus
○ C Autoimmune Henoch–Schönlein purpura
○ D Kawasaki's disease
○ E Hereditary angioneurotic oedema

126 A 4-year-old, fair-skinned red-haired boy presents to the A&E department with a long history of chronic viral illnesses associated with diarrhoea. He appears atopic with rhinorrhoea and eczema. The GP has given him four courses of antibiotics for presumed chronic otitis media. On examination, the boy is small, has a fever of 38.4°C and appears pale with small bruises over his shins. He has marked eczema over the extensor surfaces and behind the ears but no associated superinfection. He has conjunctivitis with red conjunctivae and thrush. Cardiovascular, respiratory and abdominal examination is unremarkable. The bloody diarrhoea grows *Campylobacter*. Investigations reveal a white cell count of 5.510^9 cells/l, a haemoglobin of 10.4 g/dl and a platelet count of 3010^9 cells/l, and he is lymphopenic. An immunoglobulin profile reveals a decreased level of IgM. The boy is commenced on oral erythromycin. What is the most likely diagnosis?

○ A Acute leukaemia
○ B Hyper-IgM syndrome
○ C Wiskott–Aldrich syndrome
○ D Ataxia telangiectasia
○ E X-linked agammaglobulinaemia

Extended Matching Questions

127 Theme: Complement receptor abnormalities

A CR3 complement receptor
B Alternative pathway (C5, C6, C7, C8, C9)
C C1 esterase inhibitor
D Decrease in complement receptor (CR2)
E Alternative pathway (C3 convertases)
F Alternative pathway (delay accelerating factor (DAF))
G Classical pathway (C234)
H Classical pathway, mannose-binding lectin
I C1Q, C1R, C2, C3, C4
J Properdin

Match the complement abnormalities above to the following diseases:

○ 1 Pyogenic bacterial infection B
○ 2 Glomerulonephritis-associated systemic lupus erythematosus (SLE)
○ 3 Recurrent neisserial infection
○ 4 Non-recurrent neisserial infection
○ 5 Susceptibility to infection
○ 6 Hereditary angioneurotic oedema C
○ 7 Recurrent pyogenic infections
○ 8 Renal diseases D
○ 9 Paroxysmal nocturnal haemoglobinuria J
○ 10 Pyogenic infections H

128 Theme: Human leukocyte antigens

A HLA DR2/W2, DR/W2, B8
B HLA DR3
C HLA DQW2, DR3/7
D HLA A28
E HLA B5
F HLA B27
G HLA DR5
H HLA A3/B14
I HLA B8/DR3
J HLA DR4

○ 1 Which of the above HLA associations is responsible for ankylosing
spondylitis, psoriatic arthropathy, Reiter's disease and reactive
arthritis? This reactive arthritis may occur after a gut infection with
Salmonella, Shigella, Yersinia enterocolitica or *Campylobacter* and thus
presents with bloody diarrhoea.

○ 2 Which of the above HLA associations is responsible for Behçet's disease and the arthritis of inflammatory bowel disease? Ten per cent of suffers of inflammatory bowel disease present with arthritis, and some therefore have associated ankylosing spondylitis.

○ 3 Which of the above HLA associations would be suggestive in a 3-year-old child who has been weaned on to a gluten-containing diet and subsequently suffers from abdominal protrusion, buttock-wasting and steatorrhoea, and presents with positive anti-gliadin antibodies.

129 Theme: Hypersensitivity

Match the following types of hypersensitivity with the three clinical scenarios given:

A Type I – immediate and anaphylactic hypersensitivity
B Type II – cell-bound hypersensitivity
C Type III – immune complex hypersensitivity
D Type IV – delayed T-cell hypersensitivity
E Type V – stimulatory hypersensitivity
F Type VI – killer hypersensitivity
G Type VII
H Type VIII
I Type IX
J Type X

○ 1 A 3-year-old boy is currently undergoing stem cell bone marrow transplantation due to severe combined immunodeficiency. On examination, he is found to have an erythematous maculopapular blanching rash with marked erythema of the palms of the hands and soles of the feet. He is found to have associated abdominal pain, diarrhoea and jaundice. The boy is currently in his third week of treatment, and his recent phytohaemagglutinin (PHA) test confirms that his bone marrow has grafted. You are suspicious that he may be suffering from veno-occlusive disease with an associated rejection abnormality. Which type of hypersensitivity is involved?

○ 2 A 12-year-old girl presents to the A&E department with a non-blanching purpuric rash over her lower limbs and buttocks. She is complaining of a mild abdominal pain and a virus-like illness. On examination, she is found to have red-purple purpura throughout her lower abdomen and posteriorly over her buttocks. She is also found to have swelling of the left ankle and right knee. Her investigations show her to have + + protein and + + + blood in her urine; growth has, however, proven negative. The girl's blood pressure is currently normal, as are her other observations. You wonder whether this child is suffering from meningococcaemia or a vasculitis. What type of hypersensitivity is involved?

○ 3 A child presents to the outpatient department with exophthalmia, biorbital proptosis, lid lag and loss of weight. Her thyroid function tests prove her to have a raised thyroxine (T4) level, and she is suspected of having hyperthyroidism. Which type of hypersensitivity reaction is involved?

130 Theme: Immunoglobulins

Match the following three scenarios to one of the following immunoglobulins:

A IgG
B IgM
C IgA
D IgD
E IgE

○ 1 This immunoglobulin has a molecular weight of 95 000 Da and its structure is that of a pentamer.

○ 2 This immunoglobulin is a monomer and has a molecular weight of 175 000 Da. It is often known as a B-cell surface marker.

○ 3 This immunoglobulin is involved in the placental transfer of in utero infections and is decreased in premature infants.

Infectious Diseases and Tropical Medicine

Question Frequency

Actinomycosis	0	Cat scratch disease	1
Adenovirus	3	Cerebral abcesses (adult)	4
African haemorrhagic fevers	0	Chemoprophylaxis	0
Anthrax	0	Chest X-ray	0
Antibiotic prophylaxis	0	*Chlamydia trichomatosis*	9
Antibiotics	0	Cholera – vibrio	3
Antibiotics – pharmacy	0	*Clostridium difficile*	4
Antifungal agents	0	*Clostridium difficile –*	
Aspergillosis (adult)	4	enterocolitis	2
Associations	3	*Clostridium difficile –*	
Atypical mycobacteria	1	pseudomembranous colitis	
Atypical pneumonia	1	(adult)	2
Bacillus cereus	0	*Clostridium perfringens /welchii*	1
Bacteriocidal	0	Coagulase-negative	
Bacteriostatic	0	*Staphylococcus*	0
Bacteriostatic/bacteriocidal	0	*Cryptococcus*	1
BCG	2	Cryptosporidia	2
Boils	1	*Cryptosporidium parvum*	1
Bone lesions	1	Dermatophytes	0
Borreliosis	2	Diarrhoea – infective	1
Botulism	1	Dog diseases	0
Brucellosis (adult)	6	Dysentry	0
Brucellosis – acute	0	Ebola virus	0
Campylobacter (adult)	2	Encephalitis	1
Candidiasis	1	Endotoxin	3

questions

Enterovirus	0	Malaria (adult)	7
Epiglottitis	5	Malaria – cerebral	2
Epstein–Barr virus (adult)	6	Measles (adult)	6
Familial Mediterranean fever	1	Meliodosis	0
Fever	0	Meningitis	2
Filiriid infections	0	Meningitis – *Eschericia coli*	1
Food poisoning (adult)	1	Meningitis – *Haemophilus*	2
Fucidin	0	Meningitis – meningococal	
Fungal infection (adult)	1	(adult)	3
Gentamicin toxicity	1	Meningitis – meningococcal	
Gonococcal infection (adult)	2	treatment (adult)	3
Gram-negative organisms	0	Meningitis – pneumococcal	
Gram-positive organisms	0	(adult)	2
Haemophilus influenzae	0	Meningitis – TB (adult)	6
Haemoptysis	0	Microbiology	0
Helminths	0	Molluscum contagiosum	1
Herpes – chickenpox (adult)	6	Mumps (adult)	7
Herpes – cytomegalovirus	5	*Mycobacterium intracellulare*	2
Herpes – DNA (adult)	5	*Mycoplasma pneumoniae* (adult)	7
Herpes – herpes simplex	5	Notifiable diseases	0
Herpes – varicella	1	Osteomyelitis	1
Herpes virus	5	Palm rash	0
HHV6 – roseolar infanatum	3	Parotitis – recurrent	1
Hydatid disease (adult)	2	Parvo B19 virus (adult)	4
Immunocompromised host	0	Penicillin	0
Incubation times (adult)	1	Pivampicillin	0
Indium leukocyte scanning	0	Plague	0
Infectious mononucleosis (adult)	6	Pneumococci	0
Influenza	0	*Pneumocystis carinii* pneumonia	7
Insect vectors (adult)	2	Pneumonia	0
Irritable hip	0	Polio virus	2
Jaundice	0	Pregnancy	0
Kawasaki disease (adult)	6	Protozoal infections	0
Laryngotracheobronchitis	0	Pseudo aeruginosa (adult)	1
Lassa fever	0	Q fever	0
Legionnaires' disease	1	Rabies (adult)	1
Leishmaniasis	2	Rashes	0
Leprosy	0	Rat infestations	0
Listeria monocytogenes	1	Rickettsial infections	0
Lumbar puncture	0	Rigors (adult)	1
Lyme disease (adult)	5	Rods – Gram positive	0

Rubella (adult)	5	Toxocariasis	2
Schistosomiasis	0	Toxoplasmosis (adult)	7
Septic arthritis	0	Toxoplasmosis – congenital	0
Sexually transmitted diseases	0	Tuberculosis (adult)	5
Shigella (adult)	1	Tuberculosis – drug resistance	3
Shigella encephalopathy	1	Tuberculosis – drugs (adult)	3
Spirochaetes	0	Tuberculosis – ileitis	2
Streptococcal throat infections	2	Tuberculosis – renal tract	2
Streptococcus group A	0	Typhoid fever (adult)	3
Streptococcus pneumoniae	0	Vancomycin-resistant	
Strongyloides	0	enterococci	0
Syphylis (adult)	1	Viruses	1
Tetanus (adult)	4	Weal's disease	0
Tetanus toxin	1	Whooping cough	4
Threadworm	1	Whooping cough – *Bordetella*	
Tick-borne disease	1	*pertussis*	3
Toxic shock syndrome	4	Yeast	0
Toxins (adult)	5		

questions

Multiple True/False Questions

131 With regard to chickenpox which of the following statements are true?

- A The mortality is 15 per 100 000 children aged between 1 and 11 years of age
- B It has a lower mortality rate in adults
- C It infects over 80% of people in the USA, UK and Japan
- D Intravenous aciclovir reduces clinical deterioration in children with a malignancy
- E Oral aciclovir significantly reduces the symptoms if given within 24 hours of the rash

132 Regarding toxoplasmosis, which of the following statements are true?

- A It causes a subclinical disease that may evolve into neurological disease
- B It can arise by eating unwashed vegetables
- C It can be transmitted transplacentally
- D It causes chorioretinitis
- E It is associated with congenital hydrocephalus

133 Which of the following are the recommended periods for keeping infected children out of contact with other children?

- A Chickenpox (varicella): 3 days from the time of the skin eruption
- B Fifth disease (slapped cheek syndrome): 3 days from full clinical presentation
- C Hepatitis A: 5 days in preschool children
- D Mumps: 6 days from the onset of parotitis
- E Scarlet fever: 3 days from the onset of antibiotic fever

134 Complications of influenza include which of the following?

- A Otitis media
- B Bacterial sinusitis
- C Secondary bacterial pneumonia
- D Fatigue
- E Respiratory failure

135 Which of the following statements regarding amoebiasis are true?

- A It is due an invasive trophozoite stage that can cause a colitis
- B It is invariably associated with *Entamoeba histolytica*

○ C It can give rise to amoebic liver abscesses, particularly in young men
○ D It can be a cause of rectal bleeding without diarrhoea
○ E Liver abscess can be reliably diagnosed with amoebic serology in a
suspected case

136 Which of the following statements regarding Lyme disease are true?

○ A It is due to a Gram-negative organism
○ B If untreated, it spontaneously resolves at a rate of 10–20% per year
○ C It causes neuropathies or meningitis in 15% of untreated patients
○ D It is commonly fatal
○ E Arthritis is better treated with ceftriaxone than penicillin

137 With regard to the meningococcus, which of the following statements are true?

○ A Carriage in the nasopharynx is reduced by antibiotic treatment
○ B Treatment to eradicate disease has been shown to reduce the risk of
disease
○ C Disease is increased following exposure to smoke
○ D It has its highest peak in adolescence
○ E Risk of transmission is greatest during the second week following
contact

138 With regard to acute otitis media, which of the following statements are true?

○ A The condition is reduced by chewing xylitol
○ B At day 9, the treatment failure rate is reduced by a 10-day course of
antibiotics rather than a 5-day course
○ C It is more likely to re-occur at 8–10 days than with a 10-day course of
antibiotics rather than 5 days
○ D It is more likely to be associated with reinfection at 20–30 days with a
10-day course of antibiotics rather than with a 5-day one
○ E Immediate rather than delayed antibiotic treatment leads to a
significant difference in pain scores

139 With regard to measles, which of the following statements are true?

○ A It is spread via the faecal-oral route
○ B It infects newborn children more readily than older ones
○ C It is caused by a DNA virus
○ D It has a prodromal period of 7 days
○ E It has a widespread maculopapular rash that lasts for 5–6 days

questions

140 For pulmonary tuberculosis, which of the following statements are true?

○ A A standard shortened course of 6 months of chemotherapy is associated with a higher rate of relapse than a longer (8- to 9-month) course

○ B Daily medication has a better cure rate than medication given 2 or 3 times per week

○ B Courses lasting less than 6 months are associated with an increased rate of relapse

○ D The completion of treatment is improved with repeated home visits and reminder letters than with a single reminder letter and home visit

○ E The cure/completion rate is greater with directly observed treatment versus self-treatment

141 Regarding acute tonsillitis in the UK, which of the following statements are true?

○ A It is commoner in adults

○ B It is shown by culture to be caused by β-haemolytic *Streptococcus* in 80% of cases

○ C If treated by tonsillectomy, it is associated with fewer throat infections after 2 years

○ D If treated by tonsillectomy, it is associated with fewer throat infections after 5 years

○ E It can be complicated by a peritonsillar abscess

Best of Five Questions

142 A 12-year-old boy who has returned from the Mediterranean after working on a farm presents with a chronic relapsing fever, sweating episodes and general arthralgia and anorexia. He has lost a lot of weight and is currently complaining of constipation. His previous medical history includes a week's duration of a very high fever with associated headache, arthralgia, malaise and profuse sweating. On examination, you find a very thin boy who has a papular rash throughout, swollen ankles and a left swollen elbow; the cardiovascular and respiratory examination is unremarkable. However, on palpation of the abdomen he has hepatosplenomegaly with inguinal lymphadenopathy and swollen testes. Investigations show a normal white blood cell count, but the boy's blood culture has grown a Gram-negative, non-spore-forming intracellular aerobe. What is the diagnosis?

○ A Typhoid fever
○ B *Shigella*
○ C Brucellosis
○ D Malaria
○ E Hepatitis A

143 A 2-week neonate presents with bilateral purulent conjunctivitis and difficulty breathing. On examination, the baby is found to be afebrile with normal observations and marked purulent bilateral conjunctivitis. Cardiovascular and abdominal examination is unremarkable. There is marked intercostal and subcostal recession with bilateral crepitations and expiratory wheeze. What is the diagnosis?

○ A Respiratory syncytial virus
○ B Rhinovirus
○ C Virally induced wheeze
○ D *Chlamydia trachomatis* pneumonitis
○ E Gonorrhoeal pneumonitis

144 A 14-year-old unimmunised boy presents with a high fever, malaise and bilaterally enlarged parotid glands and submandibular lymph nodes. He is also complaining of a severe headache with photophobia and neck stiffness, and has been vomiting for 24 h. Over the past 2 h, the boy's mother has noticed him to have unilateral swollen testicles. What is the diagnosis?

○ A Aseptic viral meningitis
○ B Pneumococcal meningitis
○ C Tuberculous meningitis
○ D Uncomplicated mumps
○ E Infectious mononucleosis

145 A 12-year-old girl presents with a 2-week history of fever and chronic fatigue. She is complaining of a sore throat, swollen neck glands and difficulty breathing at night. On examination, you find a thin girl with mild jaundice, marked hepatosplenomegaly and a maculopapular rash. Palatal petechiae are noticed, and marked submandibular and cervical lymphadenopathy is palpable. Investigations confirm haematuria, and blood tests depict atypical lymphocytosis, thrombocytopenia and raised levels of transaminases and alkaline phosphatase. The girl was treated with antibiotics for a sore throat. What is the diagnosis?

A Burkitt's lymphoma
B Hepatitis
C Infectious mononucleosis
D Measles
E Guillain–Barré syndrome

Extended Matching Question

146 Theme: Antibiotic actions

A Tetracycline
B Griseofulvin
C Cephalosporins
D Isoniazid
E Penicillin
F Erythromycin
G Co-trimoxazole
H Sulphonamide
I Ethambutol
J Rifampicin

For these ten drugs:

1 Which have a bactericidal effect?
2 Which have a bacteriostatic effect?
3 Which have neither?

Metabolism

Question Frequency

Acidosis – respiratory	4	Galactosaemia	6
Acute stress	0	Gangliosidoses	1
Adrenaleukodystrophy	2	Gargolysim	0
Alanine transaminase	1	Gaucher's disease	1
Alkaline phosphatase (adult)	1	Genetics	0
Alkalosis – metabolic (adult)	5	Gluconeogenesis (adult)	1
Alkalosis – respiratory	4	Glutamic aciduria	0
Amino acids	0	Glycogen storage disease	2
Ammonia	0	Glycogen storage disease –	
Amyloidosis (adult)	2	Fabry's	2
Autoimmune chronic active		Glycogen storage disease –	
hepatitis	0	type 1	2
Biotin deficiency	0	Glycogen storage disease –	
Bone disease	1	type 2	1
Cardiomyopathy	0	Glycogen storage disease –	
Cholesterol (adult)	1	type 3	0
Clinical signs	1	Glycogen storage disease –	
Conradi syndrome	2	type 4	1
Copper deficiency	0	Hartnup disease	1
Copper diseases (adult)	2	HELPP syndrome	0
Copper diseases – Menkes		Hepatomegaly	0
syndrome	0	Hepatosplenomegaly	0
Copper diseases – Wilson's		Homocystinuria (adult)	8
disease (adult)	8	Hypercholesterolaemia	0
Cystinosis	2	Hypercholesterolaemia – familial	0
Cystinuria	1	Hypercreatinaemia	0
Dehydration – hypernatraemic	1	Hyperglycaemia – non-ketotic	0
Fat absorption/metabolism		Hyperkalaemia (adult)	6
(adult)	2	Hyperlipidaemia (adult)	2
Fructosaemia	1	Hypernatraemia	4

questions

Hyperuraemia (adult)	2	Niemann–Pick disease	1
Hyperuricaemia (adult)	1	Odour	2
Hypochloridia (adult)	1	Ornithine transcarbamylase	
Hypoglycaemia	1	deficiency	1
Hypoglycaemia – ketotic	2	Pearson's syndrome	2
Hypoglycaemia – non-ketotic	3	Peroxismal disorders	2
Hypokalaemia (adult)	7	Phenylketonuria (adult)	5
Hypomagnesaemia (adult)	2	Pigmentation	1
Hyponatraemia (adult)	3	Porphyria (adult)	2
Hypophosphataemia (adult)	2	Potassium homeostasis (adult)	6
Isovaleric acidaemia	0	Pyruvate dehydrogenase	
Lactate (adult)	3	deficiency	1
Lactic acidosis	3	Refsum's disease	2
Maple syrup urine disease	1	Splenomegaly	0
MCAD	3	Tay–Sachs disease	0
Melanin production disorders	0	Tyrosinaemia	1
Mental retardation	0	Tyrosinaemia – newborn	1
Mucopolysaccaridoses	1	Urea cycle defects	1
Mucopolysaccaridoses – Hurler's		Wolman's disease	1
(adult)	2	Xanthanuria	1
Neonatal metabolic disorders	0	Zellweger's syndrome	2
Neurolipidoses	0		

Multiple True/False Questions

147 Regarding X-linked adrenoleukodystrophy, which of the following statements are true?

A It presents with progressive neurological deterioration
B It is associated with seizures
C It is diagnosed by an elevated serum phytanic acid level
D It can be stabilised by bone marrow transplantation
E It is caused by a purine disorder

148 Regarding Refsum's disease, which of the following statements are true?

A It is only seen in females
B It most often has a sudden onset
C It develops in 80% of cases in the second decade of life
D It has only a motor neuropathy
E In untreated children it commonly causes death due to cardiomyopathy

Best of Five Question

149 Chose the best statement from the five below. Patients with classic galactosaemia

A have hyperglycaemia and need treatment for their galactose-1-phosphate uridyl transferase deficiency
B can be diagnosed by red cell assay for the enzyme defect
C cannot be identified by antenatal screening
D often have excessive weight gain in the neonatal period
E present with constipation

Neonatology

Question Frequency

Abdominal distension (adult)	2	Fetal haemoglobin	0
ABO blood groups	2	Fetal lung liquid	0
ABO haemolytic disease	5	Fever	0
Air leak syndrome	0	Floppy baby	0
Anaemia	1	Gestational age	0
Apgar scores	0	Haemodynamics at birth	0
Apoptosis	0	Haemolytic disorders of newborn	2
BCG	0	Haemorrhagic disease of newborn	2
Biochemistry	0	Hearing impairment	0
Birth injuries	0	Heart failure	0
Breast milk and feeding	5	Herpes simplex infection	1
Bronchopulmonary dysplasia	4	HIE	2
Calculations	0	High-frequency oscillation	0
Choanal atresia	1	HIV	1
Chronic lung disease	0	Hyaline membrane disease	1
Circulation	0	Hydrops fetalis	4
Clotting deficiency	2	Hypoxia	0
Coagulase-negative *Staphylococcus*	0	Infection	0
Cold stress	0	Intrauterine growth retardation	4
Congenital dislocation of hip	4	Intraventricular haemorrhage	1
Congenital infections	2	Isoimmune thrombocytopenic	
Cross-infection in SCBU	0	purpura	1
Deformations/malformations	2	Kernicterus	2
Dermatology	0	LGA	0
Drugs in pregnancy	3	Lung malformation	0
Dubowitz score	0	Maternal Illness	5
Epidemiology	0	Meconium aspiration syndrome	1
Eventration of diaphragm	1	Metabolic bone disease	0
Fetal circulation	0	Metabolic disorders	1
Fetal growth	1	NEC (adult)	6

Neonatal abstinence syndrome	0	Pre-eclampsia	2
Neonatal ECG	0	Pregnancy	4
Neonatal haematology	0	Pregnancy – renal changes	1
Neonatal hyperglycaemia	0	Prematurity	0
Neonatal hypoglycaemia (adult)	5	Pulmonary haemorrhage	0
Neonatal meningitis	0	Pulmonary hypoplasia	0
Neonatal mortality rate	0	Recurrent apnoea in premature	
Neonatal polycythaemia	0	infants	0
Neonatal respiratory problems	0	Renal physiology	1
Neonatal seizures (adult)	6	Respiratory distress syndrome	
Neonatal thrombocytopenia	1	(adult)	3
Neonatal transfusion (adult)	1	Resuscitation	0
Nephrotoxic drugs	1	Retinopathy of prematurity	3
Neural tube defects	0	Rhesus haemolytic disease	1
Oligohydramnios	2	Right ventricular hypertrophy	0
Ophthalmia neonatorum (adult)	1	Septicaemia	3
Oxygen tests	0	SGA	2
Oxygen therapy	0	Sternocleidomastoid tumour	0
Perinatal asphyxia	0	Steroids in newborn	0
Periventricular haemorrhage	1	Stress	0
Periventricular leukomalacia	1	Tachycardias	0
Phototherapy	0	Tachypnoeas	1
Physiology of neonate	1	Talipes equinovarus	0
Placental transfer	1	Teratogens	3
Pneumothorax	1	Thrombocytopenia in newborn	3
Polyhydramnios	3	Umbilical cord blood	0
Post-asphyxia syndrome	1	Umbilical hernia	3
Post-haemorrhagic		Ventilation	1
hydrocephalus	1	Ventricular haemorrhage	1
Postnatal examination	1	Vitamin K	4
Postnatal problems	1	Vomiting	3
Postpartum haemorrhage	0		

Multiple True/False Questions

150 The use of antenatal steroids in anticipated preterm births is associated with which of the following?

- ○ A An increased incidence of intracranial intraventricular haemorrhage
- ○ B An increased incidence of hyaline membrane disease
- ○ C An increased neonatal mortality rate
- ○ D In combination with thyrotrophin, a reduction in neonatal mortality
- ○ E In combination with thyrotrophin, an increased number of adverse events in the pregnant woman

151 Which of the following conditions have been associated with increased nuchal thickness at prenatal scan?

- ○ A Tetralogy of Fallot
- ○ B Exomphalos
- ○ C Diaphragmatic hernia
- ○ D Noonan's syndrome
- ○ E Trisomy 21

152 Which of the following definitions are true?

- ○ A The stillbirth rate is the number of stillbirths per 1000 total births
- ○ B The perinatal mortality rate equals the number of stillbirth deaths plus the number of neonatal deaths per 1000 total deaths per year
- ○ C The infant mortality rate is the number per annum of children dying after 28 days of life and up to the end of the first year of life
- ○ D Small for gestational age is defined as being less than the 5th centile
- ○ E Extremely low birth weight is defined as less than 1500 g

153 Causes of a large-for-gestational-age baby include which of the following?

- ○ A Severe erythroblastosis
- ○ B Infant of gestational diabetic mother
- ○ C Transposition of the great vessels
- ○ D Soto's syndrome
- ○ E Hydrops fetalis

154 Avoidance of which of the following has been shown by randomised controlled trials to be effective in preventing sudden infant death syndrome?

- ○ A Prone sleeping
- ○ B Exposure to tobacco smoke
- ○ C Overheating
- ○ D Bed-sharing
- ○ E Soft sleeping surfaces

questions

Best of Five Questions

155 A female infant 2 years of age presents with delayed walking. She was born by breech delivery, and complications included oligohydramnios. Her previous medical history included hypotonia and scissoring of the legs. There is no history of myelomeningocoele, cerebral palsy or birth asphyxia. On examination, the girl is afebrile with no dysmorphism. The limbs look equal and symmetrical, but the right leg appears shorter than the left. Cardiovascular, respiratory and abdominal examination is unremarkable. Neurological examination confirms hypotonia with normal power and reflexes.

What is a possible diagnosis in the above scenario?

- A Slipped upper femoral epiphysis
- B Acute septic arthritis
- C Perthes' disease
- D Congenital dislocation of the hip
- E Acute osteomyelitis

156 You attend an urgent emergency section for a 36-week premature male infant who has presented with decreased fetal movements and an abnormal cardiotocograph. On arrival on the labour ward, you find an oedematous, pale, apnoeic infant who requires resuscitation. The mother had fetal ultrasound scans at 12, 20 and 35 weeks' gestation, at which no abnormality was noticed. The mother has a normal autoantibody, rubella, syphilis, human immunodeficiency virus and congenital infection screen. She had presented to the labour ward a week earlier with abdominal pain and bleeding, at 35 + 2 weeks' gestation. Her symptoms resolved and she was discharged home.

What is a possible cause for this baby's oedema?

- A Fetomaternal haemorrhage
- B Paroxysmal superventricular tachycardia
- C Turner's syndrome
- D Congenital infections
- E Placental chorioangioma
- F *Listeria monocytogenes*
- G Group B haemolytic *Streptococcus*

157 You review a 48-hour-old term female infant who was admitted for presumed sepsis with hypothermia and jitteriness. On examination, the infant is polycythaemic with normal symmetrical movements and tone. She is slightly jittery, with marked startling movements. The baby was born by normal vaginal delivery, weighing 1.8 kg with a length of 45 cm and a head circumference of 34.5 cm. Investigations show an initial blood glucose level of 1.0 mmol/l, haemoglobin 18.6 g/dl, white cell count 3.1 × 10⁹/l, neutrophil count 0.6 × 10⁹/l, platelet count 100 × 10⁹/l and C-reactive protein <5 mg/l, with a negative maternal and infant infection screen. The baby's mother is a smoker and suffers from anorexia nervosa. She enjoys the occasional drink.

What is the main concern regarding this neonate's admission?

- A Resistant hyperinsulinism
- B Sepsis
- C Drug withdrawal
- D Intrauterine growth retardation
- E Macrosomia

158 You review a 48-hour-old female neonate. Her initial, low blood sugar level was 1.8 mmol/l. The baby was commenced on a feeding plan and appeared to improve, but the midwives have now called you because of a marked deterioration in the baby's condition. The antenatal history is unremarkable, and the mother has no previous medical history of note. The baby was delivered weighing 4.8 kg with a length of 50.5 cm and a head circumference of 36 cm. On arrival on the antenatal ward, you find a large macrosomic baby who appears dysmorphic with prominent epicanthic folds and a large tongue. She is polycythaemic, and there is a bruise where the vitamin K injection has been given. She is jittery, with abnormal movements, and slightly tachypnoeic with an oxygen requirement of 3 l/min. She has a 2/6 pansystolic murmur at the upper left sternal edge with normal, equal and symmetrical pulses. On auscultation, there is no tracheal tug, subcostal recession or crepitation. On palpation of the abdomen, you find a swelling in the right upper quadrant that appears ballotable. Investigations show the neonate to have a blood sugar level of 1.0 mmol/l, a haemoglobin of 19.3 g/dl, a white cell count of 6.8 × 10⁹/l and a normal clotting profile. The C-reactive protein level is <5 mg/l, and the arterial blood gas shows a metabolic acidosis.

1 *A possible diagnosis is that of*

- ○ A Nesidioblastosis
- ○ B Beckwith–Wiedemann syndrome
- ○ C Down's syndrome
- ○ D Infant of diabetic mother
- ○ E Severe haemorrhagic disease of the newborn

2 *What medication should she be commenced on?*

- ○ A Intravenous glucocorticoids
- ○ B Intravenous diazoxide
- ○ C Intravenous glucocorticoids and diazoxide
- ○ D Frusemide
- ○ E Spironolactone

3 *What is the mass likely to be?*

- ○ A Neuroblastoma
- ○ B Nephroblastoma
- ○ C Medulloblastoma
- ○ D Osteosarcoma
- ○ E Ependymoma

Extended Matching Questions

159 Theme: Neonatal seizures

- A Hypoglycaemia
- B Hypoxic-ischaemic encephalopathy
- C Fifth-day fits
- D Benign familial neonatal convulsions
- E Meningitis
- F Transient hypocalcaemia
- G DiGeorge syndrome
- H Drug withdrawal
- I Hyperphenylalanaemia
- J Wilson's disease

The incidence of neonatal seizures is 6 per 1000. The aetiology is often uncertain. Match the following three scenarios to one of a possible ten diagnoses above.

- ○ 1 A 4-week male infant presents to the A&E department with abnormal movements. On examination, he is found to be happy and alert with normal tone, power and reflexes. All observations are unremarkable, with no evidence of sepsis. All investigations appear normal, and a follow-up EEG is unremarkable. The mother is concerned as he had abnormal movements as a baby and is worried that her child has epilepsy. What is the possible diagnosis?

2 You review a 1-week-old male infant who is found to have a heart murmur. Antenatal problems include maternal hyperparathyroidism, hypomagnesaemia and polycythaemia. The mother felt abnormal movements and was treated for presumed sepsis. On examination, you find a small baby with low-set ears, hypertelorism and micrognathia. He has a 2/6 ejection systolic murmur at the upper left sternal edge. The chest radiograph is unremarkable. What is the diagnosis?

3 You admit a 48-hour-old male infant to the paediatric ward for jitteriness, hypothermia, vomiting and diarrhoea. The child is the seventh sibling in a large traveller family who are well known to social services. The two eldest siblings have been on the child protection register for neglect. On examination, the baby weighs 2.6 kg with a head circumference of 35 cm and a length of 48 cm. He appears fractious and is gnawing at his fists. He is commenced on a feeding regime and given 2-hourly feeds. He continues to be agitated with sneezing and jittery movements. What is the possible diagnosis?

Nephrology

Question Frequency

A&E formulars	1	Equations	1
Acidosis – metabolic (adult)	5	Extrophy of bladder	0
Acute intestinal nephritis	1	Genetics of renal disease	0
Acute tubular necrosis	3	Gitelman's syndrome	2
Alport's syndrome	2	Glomerulonephritis	1
Amyloidosis – haemodialysis	0	Glomerulonephritis – infection	2
Anion gap	3	Glomerulonephritis –	
Antenatal renal screening	0	membranous (adult)	4
Associations (adult)	2	Glomerulonephritis –	
Balkan neuropathy	0	mesangiocapillary	1
Bartter's syndrome	4	Glomerulonephritis – post-	
Bartter's syndrome (adult)	7	streptococcal	6
Bartter's syndrome – pseudo-		Glomerulonephritis – rapidly	
Bartter's	2	progressive	1
Blood pressure	2	Glomerulosclerosis	0
Buerger's disease	4	Goodpasture's syndrome	1
Caffey's disease	1	Haematocolpos	1
Chloride metabolism	5	Haematuria	6
Complement consumption	4	Haematuria – benign familial	1
Countercurrent mechanism	1	Haematuria – macroscopic	6
Dialysis	0	Haemoglobinuria (adult)	5
Dialysis – haemodynamics (adult)	1	Haemolytic–uraemic syndrome	1
Dialysis – peritoneal (adult)	1	Henoch–Schönlein purpura	
Discolored urine (adult)	5	(adult)	5
Duplex kidneys	1	Hepatorenal syndrome	1
Ectopic kidney	1	Hypercalcuria	4
Ectopic ureter	1	Hypertension	5
Electrolyte disturbances	1	IgA nephropathy	3
Electrolyte formulars	1	Incontinence	0
Enlarged kidneys	0	Lowe's syndrome	2

questions

Multiple True/False Questions

160 Which of the following statements regarding Fanconi's syndrome are true?

- A It is due to a distal tubular failure of reabsorption
- B It is associated with galactosaemia
- C It is associated with Wilson's disease
- D It is a cause of hypokalaemia
- E It is a cause of hypoglycosuria

161 Which of the following statements regarding posterior urethral valves are true?

- A They affect females and males equally
- B They occur in 1/1 000 000 live births
- C They are a cause of in utero death
- D They can be detected by antenatal scan
- E They are a cause of renal failure in infancy

162 Which of the following statements regarding autosomal recessive polycystic kidney disease are true?

- A It is associated with biliary ectasia
- B It is due to mutations in the short arm of chromosome 6 (6p21.1–p12)
- C It is most often identified by an antenatal scan
- D It is associated with pulmonary hyperplasia
- E It may lead to portal hypertension

163 Haematuria is seen in which of the following conditions?

- A Sickle cell disease
- B Tuberculosis
- C Schistosomiasis
- D Treatment with cylophosphamide
- E Urolithiasis

164 Renal causes of renal failure include which of the following?

- A Posterior urethral valves
- B Nephrolithiasis
- C Vesicoureteric junction obstruction
- D Neuropathic bladder
- E Myoglobulinuria

165 The differential diagnosis of enuresis includes which of the following?

○ A Detrusor instability
○ B Urinary tract infection
○ C Diabetes insipidus
○ D Diabetes mellitus
○ E Neuropathic bladder

Best of Five Question

166 You review a 15-year-old male for bilateral sensorineural deafness. His deaf mother has stated that the child is having difficulty passing urine and has haematuria and proteinuria. On examination, he is a large boy with a weight >91st centile, a height <50th centile and hypertension. Cardiovascular, respiratory, abdominal and neurological examination is unremarkable. Ophthalmoscopy examination reveals cataracts and retinitis pigmentosa. Routine investigations reveal thrombocytopenia, a raised urinary creatinine level with associated hyperphosphataemia and hypocalcaemia, a normal complement level and a creatinine clearance level of 40 ml/min. A renal biopsy confirms progressive glomerular sclerosis.

Which of the following is the most likely diagnosis?

○ A Berger's IgA nephropathy
○ B Pendred's syndrome
○ C Laurence–Moon–Biedl syndrome
○ D Congenital nephrotic syndrome
○ E Alport's syndrome

167 A 9-year-old boy presents with vomiting and abdominal pain. Two months earlier, he presented with a febrile illness associated with diarrhoea, fever, jaundice and uraemia. Investigations then confirmed *Escherichia coli* O157 in the stool. This admission, he is oedematous with a left-sided facial palsy. A urine sample depicting haematuria is sent, for which the following results are found: urine osmolality 200 mosmol/l, urinary urea 100 mmol/l, urinary sodium 40 mmol/l, urine plasma: creatinine ratio 10, urine plasma: urea ratio 8 and urine plasma osmolality ratio 1; urinary sediment is present.

1   *Which of the following types of renal failure is present?*

○   A Pre-renal failure
○   B Intrinsic renal failure
○   C Post-renal failure
○   D Pre- and post-renal failure
○   E Intrinsic and post-renal failure

2   *With what initial diagnosis did the child present?*

○   A Paracetamol poisoning
○   B Acute tubular necrosis
○   C Nephrocalcinosis
○   D Haemolytic–uraemic syndrome
○   E Weil's disease

Further investigations are carried out, which show the boy to have a metabolic acidosis, hypernatraemia, hyperkalaemia, uraemia, hypocalcaemia, hyperphosphataemia, and raised creatinine and complement levels. Analysis of the blood film confirms normochromic microcyctic anaemia. An abdominal ultrasound scan shows small atrophic kidneys with dilated ureters.

3   *With the above investigations in mind and the concurrent story, what is the current cause for this child's renal failure?*

○   A Paracetamol poisoning
○   B Acute tubular necrosis
○   C Nephrocalcinosis
○   D Haemolytic–uraemic syndrome
○   E Weil's disease

Extended Matching Questions

168 Theme: Urinary discoloration

A Myoglobulinaemia
B Tetracyclines
C Phenolphthalein
D Phenylketonuria
E Laxative abuse
F Levodopa
G Isoniazid
H Iron
I Rifampicin
J Acute intravascular haemolysis

Match these aetiological causes of a discolored urine to the colour of the urine observed.

○ 1 Which **one** of the above aetiological factors causes a yellow urine?
○○ 2 Which **two** of the above aetiological factors causes a brown urine?
○ 3 Which **one** of the above aetiological factors causes a pink/orange urine?
○○○ 4 Which **three** of the above aetiological factors causes a red urine?
○ 5 Which **one** of the above aetiological factors causes a black urine?
○○ 6 Which **two** of the above aetiological factors causes a normal coloured urine?

169 Theme: Haematuria

A Haemophilia
B Benign familial haematuria
C Glucose-6-phosphatase deficiency
D Henoch–Schönlein purpura
E Tumour lysis syndrome
F Cyclophosphamide therapy
G Sickle cell disease
H Hereditary telangiectasia
I Familial nephritis
J Beetroot ingestion

○○○○○ 1 Which **five** of the above cause microscopic haematuria?
○○○○○ 2 Which **five** of the above cause macroscopic haematuria?
○ 3 Which **one** of the above causes both microscopic and macroscopic haematuria?

Neurology

Question Frequency

Abducent nerve (adult)	4	Brachial plexus lesion	0
Absent reflexes	1	Brain damage	1
Acute transverse myelitis of cord	3	Brain death	0
Aicardi syndrome	1	Brain lesions	3
Alcoholism	1	Brain tumour	0
Alpers' NDD of childhood	1	Brainstem death	0
Alzheimer's disease (adult)	2	Breath-holding attacks	1
Amaurosis fugax	0	Brown–Sequard syndrome (adult)	2
Amnesia (adult)	1	Bulbar placid palsy	0
Anatomy	0	Carotid stenosis	0
Ankle jerks	0	Carpel tunnel syndrome (adult)	1
Anterior horn cells	0	Central pontine myelinosis	0
Anterior interosseous nerve	0	Cerebellar dysfunction	1
Anterior spinal artery syndrome	0	Cerebral abscess	1
Apert's syndrome	1	Cerebral artery	1
Aqueduct stenosis	1	Cerebral calcification	1
Arnold–Chiari malformation	1	Cerebral lesions (adult)	4
Associations	1	Cerebral malformation	1
Ataxia (adult)	3	Cerebral palsy (adult)	4
Ataxia telangiectasia	3	Cerebral tumours	1
Autonomic nervous syndrome		Cerebrallar lesion (adult)	2
(adult)	2	Cerebrospinal fluid (adult)	4
Autonomic neuropathy	0	Cerebrospinal fluid leak	1
Basal ganglia disease	1	Charcot–Marie–Tooth disease	1
Batten disease	4	Cholesteatoma	1
Benign essential tremor	1	Chorea	2
Benign IC hypertension	4	Coma	1
Benign Rolandic epilepsy	3	Common peroneal nerve	2
Berry aneurysm (adult)	2	Complex partial seizures (adult)	7
Bladder dysfunction	0	Congenital central hypoventilators	1

questions

questions

Oculogyric crisis	1	Reflexes (adult)	2
Oculomotor nerve (adult)	4	Resuscitation	1
Oligoclonal bands	0	Rett's syndrome	2
Pain fibres	0	Reye's syndrome	2
Paraneoplastic syndromes	0	Rhabdomyolysis	0
Paraproteinaemia (adult)	1	Riley–Day syndrome	2
Paraproteins (adult)	1	Sagittal sinus thrombosis	1
Parinaud's syndrome	1	Sciatic nerve (adult)	3
Parkinson's disease	0	Seizures	2
Parotid swelling (adult)	2	Septo-optic dysplasia	2
Peridoxine seizures	2	Sleep	0
Peripheral neuropathy	1	Spastic paraparesis	2
Peripheral vestibular lesions	0	Spasticity	0
Persistent vegetative state	0	Speech	0
Petit mal	5	Sphingolipidosis	3
Physiology of central nervous		Spinal cord (adult)	6
system	0	Spinal muscular atrophy	2
Pick's disease	0	Stroke	3
Pinpoint meiosis	0	Sturge–Weber syndrome	1
Pituitary adenoma	1	Subacute combined degeneration	
Plagiocephaly	0	of cord	0
Posterior columns of spinal cord		Subarachnoid haemorrhage	
(adult)	5	(adult)	2
Posterior interosseous nerve	3	Subdural haematoma	2
Post-ictal state – toxicology	2	Substance P	0
Power	1	Sudden infant death syndrome	0
Preganglionic parasympathetic		Sydenham's chorea	2
fibres	1	Sympathetic nervous system	0
Prion disease (adult)	3	Syringomyelia	0
Progressive supranuclear palsy	0	Tingling	0
Proximal weakness	0	Tourette's syndrome	1
Pseudoseizures	1	Tremor	0
Ptosis	0	Trigeminal nerve (adult)	2
Pyramidal weakness	0	Trigeminal neuralgia (adult)	2
Radial nerve	4	Trinucleotide diseases	0
Radiological investigations		Trochlear nerve (adult)	2
(adult)	1	Trochlear nerve palsy (adult)	2
Radiology	1	Tuberous sclerosis (adult)	4
Ramsay Hunt syndrome	1	Tumours	2
Rasmussen's encephalitis	1	Ulnar (adult) nerve	5
Reflex anoxic seizures	3	Unilateral section posterior nerve	1

questions

Multiple True/False Questions

170 Which of the following is/are true of post-seizure management?

○ A About 1% of the UK paediatric population will have suffered a fit without fever

○ B One-third of those children suffering an afebrile fit will have a recurrent episode

○ C The population risk of a febrile fit is 12.5%

○ D The risk of epilepsy following a complex seizure is 4.1–6.0%

○ E The risk of recurrence of a febrile fit following a first seizure is 29–35%

171 Absence seizures can be reliably treated with which of the following?

○ A Ethosuximide

○ B Lamotrigine

○ C Valproate

○ D Gabapentin

○ E Cobalamin

172 Prenatally determined causes of hydrocephalus include which of the following?

○ A Aneurysm of the great vein of Galen

○ B Neonatal intraventricular haemorrhage

○ C Sex-linked stenosis of the Sylvian aqueduct

○ D Dandy–Walker syndrome

○ E Achondroplasia

173 Basal calcification is seen in which of the following conditions?

○ A Hypothyroidism

○ B Hyperparathyroidism

○ C Congenital rubella

○ D Radiotherapy

○ E Tuberous sclerosis

174 Regression in school-aged children with seizures may be due to which of the following?

○ A Wilson's disease

○ B Subacute sclerosing panencephalitis

○ C Metachromatic leukodystrophy

○ D Gaucher's disease

○ E Adrenoleukodystrophy

175 According to the International Headache Society, the criteria for the diagnosis of migraine without aura include which of the following?

○   A   A headache lasting for 1 hour
○   B   Nausea and/or vomiting, or photophobia/phonophobia
○   C   Abdominal pain lasting for at least 1 hour
○   D   A bilateral pulsating quality to the headache
○   E   Relief by physical exercise

Best of Five Question

176 16-year-old girl sitting for her A levels presents with an 8-month history of severe bilateral occipital headache associated with vomiting. During this episode, the child often feels a throbbing in her head in time with her heartbeat, which may be symmetrical. Lying in a dark room and vomiting often relieves the headache. At the time of one incidence, she is noted to have facial pallor, wetting and abdominal pain.

What is the diagnosis?

○   A   Benign postural hypertension
○   B   Migraine
○   C   Cerebral space-occupying lesion
○   D   Sinusitis
○   E   Stress due to exams

Extended Matching Question

177 Theme: Neuromuscular disorders

  A   Transverse myelitis
  B   Spinal muscular atrophy
  C   Myasthenia gravis
  D   Duchenne muscular dystrophy
  E   Myotonia congenita
  F   Guillain–Barré disease
  G   Becker's muscular dystrophy
  H   Polio
  I   Fascioscapulohumeral dystrophy
  J   Thomsen's disease

Of the ten diagnoses above, match one to each of the three clinical scenarios given.

○ 1 A 5-year-old boy presents to you with an abnormal gait and delayed walking, with delayed motor milestones. On examination, he is found to have proximal lower limb weakness and calf muscle hypertrophy. Reflexes are diminished. Examination shows a raised creatinine phosphokinase level, and an electromyograph (EMG) is diagnostic. The child has reduced IQ and has speech delay. What is the diagnosis?

○ 2 A 6-year-old boy presents with delayed motor development and an abnormal gait. The child is often found to be clumsy, often falls and presents with a tiptoe gait. He also has tight Achilles tendons. This child has normal intelligence. What is the diagnosis?

○ 3 An 18-month-old infant who has recently immigrated from Sudan presents with a painful stiff gait and delayed walking. His parents give a history of a severe fever with sore throat, general malaise and diarrhoea and vomiting. This episode was complicated by viral meningitis whereby the child became exceptionally irritable and hypertensive. On examination, you find that the child has decreased reflexes and decreased facial muscle use bilaterally. There is intermittent shallow breathing with shortness of breath. A lumbar puncture confirms a high protein level with pleocytosis and lymphocytosis and a normal glucose concentration. What is the possible diagnosis?

Oncology

Question Frequency

Acoustic neuroma	0	Malignancy – renal disease	0
Cancer – large bowel	0	Malignancy risks	1
Carcinoid syndrome (adult)	1	Mediastinal mass	0
Chemotherapy	0	Medullary cancer of thyroid	0
Craniopharyngioma	1	Metastasis	0
Ewing's sarcoma	3	Neuroblastoma	2
Germ cell tumours	0	Oncogene – ras	0
Head and neck cancer	0	Oncogenes	0
Hepatoblastoma	0	Optic glioma	1
Leukaemia – acute lymphoblastic (adult)	4	Osteosarcome (adult)	3
Leukaemia – acute myeloid (adult)	6	Pineal tumour	1
Leukaemia – chronic lymphoblastic (adult)	4	Peripheral neurectodermal tumour	0
Leukaemia – chronic myeloid (adult)	3	Retinoblastoma	2
		Rhabdomyoscarcoma	0
Leukaemia – hairy cell (adult)	3	Sacral coccygeal teratoma	0
Leukaemia – lymphoid (adult)	4	Space-occupying lesion	1
Leukoerythroblastic blood picture	1	Superior vena cava obstruction syndrome	0
Lipoma	1	Tumour lysis syndrome	2
Lymphoma – B cell	2	Tumour necrosis factor	0
Lymphoma – Burkitt's (adult)	3	Tumours	1
Lymphoma – non-Hodgkin's	2	Weight loss	0

Multiple True/False Questions

178 The good prognostic features for neuroblastoma include which of the following?

○ A Being 5 years old
○ B Stage 3
○ C Deleted chromosome 1p
○ D A high TrK level
○ E No gain of chromosome 17q

179 With regard to sacrococcygeal tumours, which of the following statements are true?

○ A 89% are malignant
○ B They are more common in boys
○ C If benign, they do not require surgical removal
○ D Urinary catecholamines should be measured
○ E They require computed tomography/magnetic resonance imaging to exclude an intraspinal involvement

Best of Five Questions

180 A 15-year-old boy presents with cervical lymphadenopathy. He complains of a 3-month history of intermittent night sweats, fever and pruritis. He has lost weight from the 50th to the 9th centile. He is currently taking ibuprofen for a painful left hip, having fallen after he stumbled at a BBQ. On examination, you find a slim young man who is pale with painless cervical lymphadenopathy. Cardiovascular, respiratory and abdominal examination is unremarkable. Investigations show a normochromic normocytic anaemia, lymphopenia, eosinophilia and a positive Coombs' test. He has a deranged alkaline phosphatase level. A differential diagnosis is given but which of the following is the most likely diagnosis?

○ A Hepatocellular carcinoma
○ B Aspergilloma
○ C Hodgkin's disease
○ D Tuberculosis
○ E Drug-induced autoimmune haemolytic anaemia

questions

181 A 3-year-old boy with Down's syndrome presents with a 2-week history of anaemia, epistaxis and bleeding gums. On examination, he is a small pale boy with multiple bruises. Investigations reveal a haemoglobin level of 4.2 g/dl, a white count of 3.3×10^9 cells/l, a lymphocyte count of 62.4×10^9 cells/l and a platelet count of 80×10^9 cells/l. A blood film depicts promyelocytes, myelocytes and myelomonocytic cells. Auer rods and agranular neutrophils are also noted. What is the most likely diagnosis?

○ A Iron deficiency anaemia
○ B Anaemia of chronic disease
○ C Acute myeloid leukaemia (AML)
○ D Acute lymphocytic leukaemia (ALL)
○ E Chronic myeloid leukaemia (CML)

Ophthalmology

Question Frequency

Multiple True/False Questions

182 Which of the following conditions may present with concomitant strabismus?

- ○ A Retinoblastoma
- ○ B Optic nerve hypoplasia
- ○ C Bilateral cataracts
- ○ D VIII nerve cranial palsy
- ○ E Optic atrophy

183 Acquired nystagmus may be due to which of the following?

- ○ A A suprasellar tumour
- ○ B Batten disease
- ○ C Neurolipidoses
- ○ D Peroxisomal disorders
- ○ E A posterior fossa mass

Best of Five Question

184 An 8-year-old girl presents with a 2-week history of an erythematous painful eye. She complains of blurred vision and photophobia. Her mother has noticed an increase in her tears. The GP wondered whether there was a periumbal flush next to the limbus. On examination, you find a hypopyon, a muddy iris with papillary meiosis and corneal injection.

What is the possible diagnosis here?

- ○ A Glaucoma
- ○ B Corneal opacity
- ○ C Cataract
- ○ D Dislocated lens
- ○ E Uveitis

Extended Matching Questions

185 Theme: Ophthalmoscopy

A Trauma to the cornea
B Congenital rubella
C Glaucoma
D TORCH infections
E Insulin-dependent diabetes mellitus
F Hunter's syndrome
G Herpes simplex infection
H Tuberous sclerosis
I Chronic keratitis
J Hurler's syndrome

Of the ten diseases above, which match the following three clinical scenarios?

○○○○ 1 Which **four** may present with corneal opacities?
○○○○ 2 Which **four** may present with corneal clouding?
　　○ 3 Which **one** may present with a clear cornea?

186 Theme: Pupillary signs

A Severe hypoxia
B Inner brain damage
C Barbiturate usage
D Metabolic conditions
E Midbrain lesion
F Tentorial herniation
G Post-seizure activity
H Opiate usage
I Medullary lesion
J Hypothermia

Which of the ten aetiological factors above match the three pupillary signs described below?

○○○ 1 Which **three** of the above factors would cause a fixed, pinpoint pupil?
○○○○○ 2 Which **five** of the above factors would cause a fixed dilated pupil?
　　○ 3 Which **one** of the above factors would cause a unilateral dilated pupil?

187 Theme: Uveitis

    A Crohn's disease
    B Whipple's disease
    C Ulcerative colitis
    D Insulin-dependent diabetes mellitus
    E Toxocariasis
    F Toxoplasmosis
    G Acute rheumatic fever
    H Sarcoidosis
    I   Behçet's disease
    J Rheumatoid arthritis

Of these ten causes of uveitis, which correspond to the following three clinical scenarios?

◯◯ 1 Which **two** infections cause uveitis?
◯◯ 2 Which **two** musculoskeletal diseases cause uveitis?
◯◯ 3 Which **two** inflammatory disorders *commonly* cause uveitis?

188 Theme: Visual field disorders

    A Optic nerve dysfunction
    B Homonymous hemianopia
    C Optic tract dysfunction
    D Bitemporal hemianopia
    E Bitemporal superior quadrantanopia
    F Bitemporal inferior quadrantanopia
    G Temporal superior lobe radiation dysfunction
    H Parietal inferior lobe radiation dysfunction
    I   Lateral geniculate body dysfunction
    J Disorders of the pupillary response

Of the ten visual field disorders in the list above, match the relevant ones to the three clinical scenarios below.

◯◯ 1 A 12-year-old boy attends the clinic with a diagnosis of a pituitary tumour. He initially presented to his GP with tunnel vision and impaired lateral peripheral vision. Which **two** of the above defects does he present with?

◯◯ 2 A 10-year-old girl presents to the outpatient clinic with the diagnosis of a suprasellar tumour. She also presents with tunnel vision, impaired tunnel vision and impaired lateral peripheral vision. Which **two** of the above visual defects does she have?

  ◯ 3 A 16-year-old girl presents to the A&E department after a trial driving lesson with unilateral blindness with impaired visual acuity. She is unable to read the colour charts and therefore has a defect in colour vision. She is diagnosed with a demyelinating papillitis and is subsequently investigated for multiple sclerosis. Which **one** of the above ten visual field defects does she suffer from?

189 Theme: Tunnel vision and papilloedema

A Hard exudates
B Retinal vein thromboses
C Retinitis pigmentosa
D Severe myopia
E Malignant hypertension
F Glaucoma
G Tuberculous meningitis
H Subdural haematoma and bleed
I Scotoma
J Optic atrophy

Match the ten aetiological causes of tunnel vision and papilloedema to the following three clinical scenarios.

○○○ 1 A child presents to the clinic with tunnel vision. Which **three** of the above are likely aetiological factors?

○○○○○ 2 A child presents to the paediatric outpatient department with papilloedema. Which **five** of the above aetiological factors may be responsible for this?

○ 3 A child presents to the paediatric outpatient clinic with both tunnel vision and papilloedema. Which **one** of the above aetiological factors is plausible?

Psychiatry

Question Frequency

Abdominal pain – non-organic (adult)	3	Delusions (adult)	1
Abuse – alcohol (adult)	2	Dementia	0
Abuse – drug	0	Dementia – pseudo	0
Abuse – non-accidental injury	1	Depression	1
Abuse – physical	3	Depression – childhood	2
Abuse – sexual	3	Educational underachievement	0
Agoraphobia	0	Electroconvulsive therapy	1
Alcohol withdrawal (adult)	3	Emotional disorders	0
Anorexia nervosa (adult)	8	Emotional neglect (adult)	1
Asperger's syndrome	2	Encopresis	0
Associations	0	Enuresis	2
Attention deficit disorder (adult)	4	Enuresis – nocturnal (adult)	3
Attention deficit hyperactivity disorder	1	Epidemiology	0
		Epilepsy	0
Autism (adult)	5	Glue-sniffing	0
Behavioural disorders	2	Habit disorders	0
Bereavement	0	Hallucinations – visual (adult)	1
Bipolar illness	0	Hyperkinetic disorder (adult)	3
Bulimia nervosa (adult)	5	Hypomania	0
Child protection	0	Hysterical paraplegia	1
Children Act 1989	0	Injury – ageing	0
Chronic fatigue syndrome	0	Insomnia (adult)	3
Compensation neurosis	0	Korsakoff's syndrome	0
Compulsive water-drinking (adult)	1	Language	3
		Language disorders	1
Conduct disorders	0	Learning disabilities (adult)	4
Conversion somatisation	1	Mania (adult)	2
Delerium	0	Mental handicap (adult)	2
		Mental Health Act	0

Mental illness (adult)	4	Psychosis	0
Mental retardation (adult)	2	Puerperal psychosis	1
Methylphenidate hydrochloride		Schizophrenia	4
toxicity	1	School refusal	3
Munchausen's-by-proxy (adult)	5	Self-harm	0
Neurotic grief reaction	0	Sleep patterns (adult)	2
Obsessional neurosis (adult)	4	Specific reading disorder	0
Organic disease (adult)	3	Strabismus	0
Panic attack	0	Sudden infant death syndrome	2
Paranoid psychosis	0	Suicide	0
Parasuicide (adult)	2	Tardive dyskinesia	0
Pharmacy	0	Toddlers – feeding problems	0
Phobic states (adult)	2	Toe-walking	1
Prevalence of psychiatric		Tricyclic antidepressants	0
disorder	1	Truancy	0
Psychiatry and systemic disease	1	Twin studies	0
Psychology referral	1		

Multiple True/False Questions

190 Risk characteristics of abused children and their families include which of the following?

- ○ A Large-for-dates baby
- ○ B Low parental self-esteem
- ○ C Large family
- ○ D Separation from the mother in the neonatal period
- ○ E Product of an unwanted pregnancy

191 The following percentages indicate the frequency of behavioural problems in 4-year-old children. Which are correct?

- ○ A Temper tantrums – 20%
- ○ B Poor relationships with peers – 35%
- ○ C Regular soiling – 8%
- ○ D Poor concentration – 15%
- ○ E Poor appetite – 3%

192 Which of the following statements regarding childhood autism is true?

- ○ A It is three times more common in girls
- ○ B It has a frequency of 150/100 000 children
- ○ C It is associated with normal language development
- ○ D It is associated with an IQ >120 in 70% of autistic children
- ○ E It is associated with a lack of empathy

193 Major criteria for the definition of chronic fatigue syndrome (CFS) as given by the Centers for Disease Control and Prevention include which of the following?

- ○ A The absence of depression
- ○ B Fatigue reducing activity to 75% of the patient's premorbid activity for at least 6 months
- ○ C Fatigue reducing activity to 50% of the patient's premorbid activity for at least 6 months
- ○ D Symptoms explained by infection with infectious mononucleosis
- ○ E A peak onset at 12–14 years of age

questions

194 A 12-year-old boy presents with a deterioration in concentration and attention. His parents have found him to be clumsy and restless, and he fidgets when spoken to. He is easily distracted and unable to complete one task. His literacy and cognitive function is normal, and he gives good eye contact. The boy is unable to wait his turn in line for exercises, and he is moody and aggressive in his behaviour. There is no suggestion of truancy or school refusal.

1   *What would you request to enable a possible diagnosis?*

- A   A school visit by the health visitor
- B   An appointment at home to monitor family circumstances and parenting skills
- C   A Statement for Education
- D   A Connors' Teachers Rating School Questionnaire
- E   A dietetic opinion

2   *With the above request in mind, what is the likely diagnosis?*

- A   A normal variant of difficult behaviour
- B   A conduct disorder
- C   An emotional disorder
- D   Attention deficit hyperactivity disorder (ADHD)
- E   Autistic spectrum disorder

3   *With the above diagnosis in mind, what is the pharmacological treatment?*

- A   Behaviour modification programme
- B   Dexamphetamine
- C   Methylphenidate hydrochloride
- D   Speech and language therapy
- E   Referral to a school for moderate learning difficulties

195 A 6-year-old girl presents with a long standing history of intermittent fevers, drowsiness and poor weight gain. She has been fully investigated for failure to thrive as she has attended with dehydration and hypoglycaemia secondary to vomiting and diarrhoea. Her mother gives many different histories but is adamant that the child suffers from recurrent fevers with associated vomiting, haematemesis and diarrhoea. The girl's blood results show the following levels: sodium 210 mmol/l, potassium 2.9 mmol/l, glucose 1.6 mmol/l, urea 9.3 mmol/l and creatinine 64 μmol/l. She has been hospitalised for a total of 14 months. The parents want a diagnosis.

1   *What is the likely diagnosis?*

○   A   Somatisation
○   B   Malingering
○   C   Munchausen by proxy
○   D   Hysterical conversion disorder
○   E   Inflammatory bowel disease

2   *Of the following aetiological factors, which is the most plausible?*

○   A   Poisoning
○   B   Insulin administration
○   C   Sexual abuse
○   D   Physical abuse
○   E   Abuse of neglect

3   *Which of the following clues would make you suspect the diagnosis?*

○   A   Persistent recurrent illness that cannot be explained
○   B   Investigatory results that do not correlate with clinical history or examination
○   C   The parent always being present at times of abnormality
○   D   The treatment appearing to be ineffective
○   E   All of the above

Extended Matching Questions

196 Theme: Behaviour disorders

List A
A   Behaviour disorder
B   Emotional disorder
C   Bulimia nervosa
D   Conduct disorder
E   Anorexia nervosa

a)   1   For each of the following descriptions, select the correct behaviour disorder from the list above. Each option may be used once, more than once or not at all.

○   A preoccupation with eating that causes overeating and obesity
○   A preoccupation with eating that causes loss of weight and starvation
○   A family history of maternal depression, emotional neglect and child abuse
○   A family history of a full-time working mother, a sibling with cystic fibrosis or previous residential care in a home

○ The resultant anxiety is counteracted by the vomiting and purging of food substances

○ The resultant anxiety is counteracted by vomiting and food refusal

○ The desire to eat liquidised foods

○ The fear of fatness and a distorted body image

○ The need to use laxatives, diuretics and stimulatory medication

○ Comfort eating leads to guilt and finally depression

b) *Match the following scenarios to the list of diagnoses in List A.*

○ 1 A meticulous and tidy 17-year-old female presents with vomiting, dehydration and general malaise. She has previously been well, with no preceding illness. On examination, she is afebrile and has dental caries, a parotid enlargement and a positive Russell's sign. Her weight is on the 50th centile and she has reached stage 5 of puberty. Results show hypokalaemia, uraemia and hypernatraemia. She has a normal lipid and hormone profile. What is the diagnosis?

○ 2 A slim, unkempt 17-year-old female presents with vomiting, dehydration, general malaise and tiredness. She complains of secondary amenorrhoea. On examination, she is afebrile and has dental caries and a positive Russell's sign. Her weight is <0.4th centile, and her puberty status is delayed in that she is amenorrhoeic. She is hypernatraemic, hypokalaemic and uraemic, and has hypochromic normocytic anaemia. She has deranged hormone and lipid profiles. What is her diagnosis?

○ 3 A 4-year-old boy presents with severe tantrums, sleep disturbance, enuresis, encopresis and is a faddy eater. What is the diagnosis?

197 Theme: Learning difficulty

    A Hypothyroidism
    B Language delay
    C Depression
    D Huntington's chorea
    E Conduct disorder
    F Insulinoma
    G Bullying
    H Vitamin B12 deficiency
    I Attention deficit hyperactivity disorder (ADHD)
    J Child sexual abuse

Match the three clinical statements below to the following ten causes of learning difficulty.

○○○ 1 A 12-year-old girl presents with regression of educational achievement. There have been some concerns with respect to her social interaction towards her friends in the class, and Social Services have recently been involved because of possible domestic violence. Which **three** causes from the list above may be associated confounding factors?

○○○ 2 A 7-year-old boy presents with regression in his reading and writing skills. He is clumsy, agitated, moody and aggressive. He is distracted in class and unable to wait his turn. Of the above conditions, which **three** causes may be confounding factors?

○○○○ 3 A 10-year-old boy presents with intellectual deterioration and developmental regression. There has been a gradual deterioration in all aspects, including reading, writing and mathematical and scientific subjects. From the list above, which **four** confounding factors may be relevant?

198 Theme: Odd behaviour

A Conduct disorder
B Schizophrenia
C Obsessional neuroses
D Neurotic mother
E Munchausen's by proxy

A 16-year-old boy attends with an 18-month history of impaired concentration, poor memory and disturbed sleep. He is irritable and restless with a non-intentional tremor and is intermittently sweaty with palpitations. He suffers from anxiety, and there are occasions on which he begins to hyperventilate and needs to return home immediately to check whether the iron is switched off. This is becoming a disturbing habit that is causing problems socially.

1 Of the following five diagnoses above, which is most plausible?

○ A Paraesthesia
○ B Diarrhoea
○ C Neck pain
○ D Dry mouth
○ E Dizziness
○ F Tension headache
○ G Panic attacks
○ H Palpitations and sweating
○ I Faintness
○ J Failure of erection

Of the ten clinical symptoms precipitated by anxiety above, which would fit the three questions below?

○○○○ 2 Autonomic activity is associated with which **four** of the above disorders?

○○○○○ 3 Hyperventilation is often associated with which **five** of the above clinical symptoms?

○○ 4 Increased smooth muscle tone is associated with which **two** of the above clinical symptoms?

Respiratory Medicine

Question Frequency

Acute life threatening event	0	Cavitating lung lesions (adult)	3
Acute respiratory distress		Chemo-related lung disease	0
syndrome	0	Cheyne–Stokes respiration	0
AIDS	0	Chronic interstitial lung disease	
Airway obstruction	0	(adult)	1
Alpha protease inhibitor	3	Churg–Strauss syndrome	0
Alveolar macrophage	0	Clubbing	0
Anatomy	1	Clubbing (adult)	1
Antioxidant defences	0	Compliance	0
α_1-Antitrypsin deficiency	6	Congenital central hypoventilation	
Arterial blood	2	syndrome	1
Arterial blood gas	2	Congenital lobar emphysema	0
Asbestosis	0	Congenital lung disease	0
Asphyxia	1	Congenital pulmonary	
Associations (adult)	1	lymphangectasia	0
Asthma	6	Cough	1
Asthma – environment	6	Crackles at lung bases	2
Atelectasis	1	Croup	2
Basic science	0	Cystic adenomatoid malformation	0
Bronchial liability index	0	Cystic fibrosis (adult)	11
Bronchiectasis (adult)	8	Cystic fibrosis – CFTR	2
Bronchoalveolar lavage	0	Cystic fibrosis – radiology	0
Bronchogenic cysts	0	Diaphragmatic hernia	2
Bronchopulmonary dysplasia	0	Disassociation curve (adult)	5
Bronchoscopy	1	Drowning	0
Capillary alveolar block	1	Eaton–Lambert syndrome	0
Carbon dioxide	0	Emphysema (adult)	3
Carbon monoxide transfer factor		Exercise physiology	0
(TLCO)	3	Fibrosing alveolitis (adult)	3
Carcinoma of bronchus	0	Fibrosing alveolitis – cryptogenic	1

questions

Finger clubbing	0	Peak expiratory flow rate	1
Flow–volume loops	2	Phrenic nerve	0
Foreign body	2	Physiology (adult)	2
Granulomatosis lung disease	0	Pleural calcification	0
Haemoptysis	0	Pleural effusions (adult)	5
Haemorrhagic pulmonary		Pneumoconiosis	0
oedema	2	Pneumonia (adult)	6
Haemosiderosis	1	Pneumothorax	4
Haemosiderosis – primary	1	Pneumothorax radiology	1
Harrison's sulcus	1	Poland's syndrome	0
Hemidiaphragm	1	Potter's syndrome	1
High-altitude living	0	Psittacosis	0
Hyaline membrane disease	0	Pulmonary alveolar proteinosis	1
Hypercarbia/hypocarbia	0	Pulmonary embolism	5
Hyperexpansion	0	Pulmonary eosinophilia	0
Hypertrophic osteopathy	0	Pulmonary fibrosis	0
Hypoxia	1	Pulmonary function (adult)	2
Inhalation	0	Pulmonary function tests (adult)	5
Laryngomalacia	0	Pulmonary hypertension	1
Laws of science	0	Pulmonary hypoplasia	0
Left isomerism	0	Pulmonary nodule (adult)	0
Legionnaires' disease (adult)	1	Pulmonary parasitic infection	1
Lobar sequestration	0	Pulmonary veno-occlusive	
Lung defects	2	disease	0
Lung growth disorders	0	Pulse oximetry	1
Lymphocytic interstitial		Reflux index	0
pneumonitis (adult)	1	Respiratory cilia	0
Mechanical ventilation	0	Respiratory failure (adult)	5
Nasal continuous positive airway		Respiratory failure – type 1	
pressure (CPAP)	1	(adult)	6
Nasal intermittent positive airway		Respiratory failure – type 2	1
pressure (IPPV)	0	Respiratory function	1
Nasal obstruction	0	Respiratory muscle disease	0
Neurenteric cyst	1	Respiratory tract infections	0
Nitric oxide (adult)	7	Sarcoidosis (adult)	2
Nocturnal hypoxaemia	0	Scimitar syndrome	0
Obstructive sleep apnoea (adult)	5	Sleep study	0
Occupational exposure (adult)	1	Smoking	0
Oesophagus and lung	0	Stridor (adult)	4
Oxygen therapy	0	Stridor – acute	0
Oxygen therapy – long term (adult)	1	Stridor – chronic	0

questions

questions

Multiple True/False Questions

199 Which of the following statements regarding sweat tests is correct?

○ A They cannot be performed on subjects taking flucloxacillin
○ B They require 100 mg of sweat to be collected
○ C They need for be carried out for a minimum of 1 hour
○ D They require sweat potassium, sodium and osmolality to be measured
○ E They can be associated with burns to the skin if unbuffered solutions are used

200 Causes of central hypoventilation include which of the following?

○ A Arnold–Chiari syndrome
○ B Familial dysautonomia
○ C Hypothyroidism
○ D Myasthenia gravis
○ E Hyperthermia

201 Cystic fibrosis may present with which of the following?

○ A Atypical gastro-oesphageal reflux
○ B Tall stature
○ C Hyperproteinaemia
○ D Nasal polyps
○ E Asthma resistant to treatment

202 Which of the following statements regarding upper airway obstruction due to epiglottis is correct?

○ A It is best treated with nebulised steroids
○ B It is associated with hypothermia
○ C It is common in the UK population
○ D It may have a sudden onset
○ E It requires a lateral X-ray of the neck

Best of Five Question

203 Choose the best statement from the five given below. The individual with the highest risk factors for pulmonary arterial hypertension is:

○ A a woman with human immunodeficiency virus (HIV) infection taking amphetamines
○ B an obese 40-year-old man who smokes
○ C a man on antidepressant medication
○ D a woman taking the oral contraceptive pill
○ E a man with sickle cell disease

204 A 4-year-old boy presents with global developmental delay. He has Prader–Willi syndrome, obesity, nocturnal enuresis, difficult behaviour as well as poor attention, listening, reading and concentration skills in class. He snores at night and has choking-like episodes when asleep. He often complains of early morning headache, sweating and intermittent fevers. He often falls asleep in class. Results from routine investigations have included normal electrolyte levels, full blood count, pH study and videofluoroscopy. An ECG has shown right ventricular hypertrophy.

1 *What investigation is most likely to give a diagnosis?*

○ A Polysonography
○ B Computed tomography
○ C Magnetic resonance imaging
○ D Sleep study
○ E Audiovisual monitoring

2 *What is the likely diagnosis?*

○ A Periodic limb movement disorder
○ B Restless legs syndrome
○ C Narcolepsy
○ D Central hyperventilation syndrome
○ E Obstructive sleep apnoea

205 An 8-year-old girl presents with a 3-week history of an intermittent fever and coryzal illness. She has had tachypnoea with a productive cough and wheeze for 10 days, is complaining of right upper quadrant abdominal pain and is anorexic. On examination, she is a slim child who is anaemic, febrile and short of breath. She has a mild tracheal tug with minimal subcostal and intercostal recession. On auscultation, she has decreased lung expansion and breath sounds with increased bronchial breathing and vocal/tactile fremitus on the right side of her chest.

questions

questions

1   The differential diagnosis is given below. What is the likely cause for her fever?

○   A Community-acquired pneumonia
○   B Hospital-acquired pneumonia
○   C Asthma
○   D Atypical pneumonia
○   E Hepatitis

2   Her chest radiograph confirms your findings. The radiograph shows that the lung is well expanded and penetrated with no evidence of cysts, pneumatocoeles, effusions or pneumothorax. What is the most likely organism?

○   A *Klebsiella*
○   B *Chlamydia psittaci* (psittacosis)
○   C *Mycoplasma*
○   D *Streptococcus pneumoniae*
○   E *Mycobacterium tuberculosis*

3   What is the appropriate treatment?

○   A Erythromycin
○   B Tetracycline
○   C Azithromycin
○   D Amphotericin
○   E Penicillin

206 An obese16-year-old girl presents with acute shortness of breath. She has recently been in bed with a flu-like illness. On examination, you find a large girl who is tachypnoeic, cyanosed and febrile. She has an intermittent dry cough and is complaining of left-sided chest pain. The girl appears slightly confused and delirious. She is slightly cyanosed with a tracheal tug and mild subcostal recession. Her heart sounds reveal an irregular heart rate in a gallop rhythm. On auscultation, she has a pleural rub and rhonchi over the left lower zone with basal crepitations. Her chest radiograph is normal. An arterial blood gas shows respiratory alkalosis.

1   What investigation is most likely to be carried out next to provide a diagnosis?

○   A ECG
○   B Ventilation–perfusion scan
○   C Spiral computed tomography (CT) scan
○   D Full blood count
○   E Sputum sample

2   *What is the likely diagnosis?*

○   A   Community-acquired pneumonia
○   B   Hospital-acquired pneumonia
○   C   Pulmonary embolism
○   D   Empyema
○   E   Pneumothorax

Extended Matching Questions

207 Theme: Pleural effusion

A   Pneumoconiosis
B   Pneumonia
C   Nephrotic syndrome
D   Dilated cardiomyopathy
E   Tuberculosis
F   Nephritic syndrome
G   Constrictive pericarditis
H   Peritoneal dialysis fluid
I   Hodgkin's disease

An 8-year-old boy post-renal transplantation is reviewed in the renal clinic with shortness of breath, fever, chest pain and a pleural effusion on his chest radiograph.

○○○ 1   Which **three** of the ten above diagnoses are plausible?
  ○ 2   Which **one** of the above diagnoses is indicative of a haemorrhagic pleural effusion?
  ○ 3   Which **one** of the above diagnoses is associated with a straw-coloured pleural effusion?

208 Theme: Transfer factor

A   Fever and increased metabolism
B   Anaemia
C   Pulmonary embolism
D   Polycythaemia
E   Empyema
F   Pulmonary hypertension
G   Increased pulmonary and capillary blood flow
H   Pneumonectomy
I   Pulmonary haemorrhage
J   Athletes and increased exercise

Which of these ten clinical presentations are associated with the three scenarios below?

○○○○○○ 1 A 5-year-old boy presents to you with a respiratory illness, his transfer factor level being increased. Which **six** of the above ten diagnoses might he have?

○○○○○ 2 A 6-year-old girl presents to you with a respiratory illness and a decreased transfer factor. Which **five** of the above clinical diagnoses might be responsible?

○ 3 Which **one** of the above disorders may show a high or a low transfer factor?

Rheumatology

Question Frequency

Achondroplasia (adult)	4	Chondrocalcinosis	1
Amniotic bands	1	Craniocleidodysostosis	1
Anatomy	0	Dermatomyositis (adult)	3
Ankylosing spondylitis (adult)	4	Developmental dyplasia of hip	1
Arthralgia	1	Diaphyseal achalasia	1
Arthritis – gonococcal	0	Dwarfism	2
Arthritis – Juvenile Chronic Arthritis (JCA)	6	Dysplasia	0
		Ellis–van Creveld syndrome	1
Arthritis – pauciarticular	5	Endnocrinopathies	1
Arthritis – polyarticular	5	Epiphyses	2
Arthritis – psoriatic (adult)	3	Extractable nuclear antigen	1
Arthritis – reactive (adult)	3	Fat embolism (adult)	1
Arthritis – rheumatoid (adult)	6	Felty's syndrome	1
Arthritis – septic (adult)	2	Forrester's disease	0
Arthritis – systemic JCA	1	Frontal bossing (adult)	2
Arthrogryposis congenita	1	Gout (adult)	1
Arthrogryposis multiplex congenita	1	Hemihypertrophy	1
		Hypochondroplasia	2
Arthropathies	2	Intra-articular steroid injection	0
Arthropathy – reactive	2	Joint hypermobility	0
Aseptic necrosis	1	Joint pain	1
Asphyxiating thoracic dystrophy	2	Joints	1
Associations (adult)	2	Klippel–Feil anomaly	1
Autoantibodies	2	Kyphoscoliosis (adult)	2
Avascular necrosis of bone	2	Madelung's deformity of wrist	1
Behçet's disease	5	Mixed connective tissue diseases	0
Biology of joint	0	Ollier's disease	1
Bone cysts	1	Osteoarthritis (adult)	2
Bowed tibia (adult)	2	Osteogenesis imperfecta	2
Charcot's joints	0	Osteomalacia	1

questions

Osteopetrosis	1	Slipped femoral epiphysis	3
Osteoporosis (adult)	3	Spondyloarthropathies	0
Paget's disease (adult)	2	Synovial fluid	1
Painful limp	1	Systemic lupus erythematosus	
Perthes' disease	1	(adult)	10
Phosphate metabolism disorders	0	Systemic lupus erythematosus –	
Polyarteritis nodosa	1	anticoagulant	2
Polymyalgia rheumatica	0	Systemic lupus erythematosus –	
Polymyositis	1	drug induced (adult)	8
Pseudoarthrosis	1	Systemic lupus erythematosus –	
Radiological bone erosions		lupus nephritis	2
(adult)	3	Systemic lupus erythematosus –	
Radiology	1	neonatal lupus	6
Raynaud's phenomenon	2	Systemic sclerosis (adult)	3
Reflex sympathetic dystrophy		Takayasu's arteritis (adult)	3
syndrome	2	Temporal arteritis	1
Reiter's disease (adult)	2	Vasculitis (adult)	4
Rheumatoid factor	0	Vasculitis – Churg–Strauss	1
Sacroileitis	0	Waldenström's	
Scleroderma	0	macroglobulinaemia	0
Scoliosis	1	Wegener's granulomatosis	1
Sjögren's sydrome	0		

Multiple True/False Questions

209 The criteria for Kawasaki disease include which of the following?

- A Fever
- B Coronary aneurysm
- C Elevated C-reactive protein level
- D Diffuse, non-specific rash
- E An enlarged inguinal lymph gland

210 In a child with discitis, which of the following are true?

- A The child may present by limping
- B The child may refuse to walk
- C Culture of the disc tissue is required
- D The radiograph may show disc space narrowing
- E The child will respond poorly to antibiotic therapy

211 A monoarthritis may be seen in which of the following conditions?

- A Sickle cell disease
- B Diabetes mellitus
- C After dysentery
- D Acute leukaemia
- E After meningococcal disease

212 Regarding Perthes' disease, which of the following statements are true?

- A It is seen most frequently in teenagers
- B It is more common in girls
- C It is caused by excessive exercise
- D It requires operative treatment in 98% of cases
- E It is bilateral in 78% of patients

Best of Five Questions

213 A 16-year-old male Caucasian presents with left hip, right knee and lower lumbar vertebral pain that is relieved by exercise. Cardiovascular examination depicts a 2/6 pansystolic murmur in diastole. Neurologically, the boy is found to have normal tone but decreased ankle jerks. Musculoskeletal examination appears unremarkable. Investigations show a raised alphafetoprotein level, normal rheumatoid factor and a normal autoantibody screen. Radiology reveals square vertebrae with a fused sacroiliac joint. There is increased soft tissue swelling of the ligaments, which are calcified.

What is the possible diagnosis in this case?

○ A Rheumatoid arthritis
○ B Ankylosing spondylitis
○ C Osteoarthritis
○ D Septic arthritis
○ E Dermatomyositis

214 A 16-year-old boy attends with painful knees, ankle and wrists. He has suffered from early morning headaches and appears often confused and delirious. He has had a 4-day history of nausea and abdominal pain associated with diarrhoea and rectal bleeding. On examination, there are papules and pustules over his shins. He has oral and genital ulceration with a tender abdomen in the right iliac fossa. Fundoscopy reveals anterior uveitis. Radiological investigations show non-erosive lesions within the bones. Serum blood samples reveal a raised erythrocyte sedimentation rate and C-reactive protein level, as well as a leukocytosis. A lumbar puncture shows a raised protein level with multiple polymorphonucleocytes and mononuclear cells, and a normal glucose level.

Which of the human leukocyte antigen (HLA) results is likely to be found in the case above?

○ A HLA DRW2
○ B HLA B27
○ C HLA B5
○ D HLA B35
○ E HLA DQW2

215 A 14-year-old girl presents with a toenail infection. She was started on an antifungal medication but has subsequently developed a painful ankle and an erythematous facial rash. Routine investigations are all normal. An autoantibody profile showed the following results:

• **Positive anti-single-stranded DNA antibody**
• **Positive ANA antibody**
• **Negative rheumatoid factor antibody**
• **Positive antihistone antibody**
• **Positive anticardiolipin antibody**

Which diagnosis is suggestive for the case above?

○ A Dermatomyositis
○ B Lupus anticoagulant syndrome
○ C Systemic lupus erythematosus (SLE)
○ D Lupus nephritis
○ E Drug-induced lupus (DIL)

216 A male neonate presents with asymmetrical growth retardation. Dysmorphic features include frontal bossing, a depressed nasal bridge, hypoplastic maxillae, broad and short limbs, a trident hand deformity and constrictive thoracic dystrophy. On examination, he has a normal head circumference. A skeletal survey shows small, square iliac crests with flat horizontal acetabular roofs, a champagne glass appearance of the pelvic rim, rhizomelic limb shortening and abnormal lumbar, sacral and skull X-rays. Ossification is normal.

Which is the most likely diagnosis?

○ A Achondrogenesis
○ B Thanatophoric dysplasia
○ C Ellis–van Creveld syndrome
○ D Hypochondroplasia
○ E Achondroplasia

217 A 12-year-old Caucasian girl presents with symmetrically painful wrists. She has had intermittent episodes of malaise and fever associated with arthralgia and myalgia. Over the past 6 months, she has progressively lost weight and suffered from alopecia. Recently, on returning from the beach, she was found to have a facial and body rash. Examination is normal. Investigations show the girl to have a hypochromic, normocytic anaemia, thrombocytopenia, lymphopenia, decreased C3 and C4 levels and raised immunoglobulins. The autoantibody profile shows positivity to rheumatoid factor, anticardiolipin antibodies, anti-double-stranded DNA, anti-Ro–La, antineutrophil cytoplasmic antibody and anti-smooth muscle antibody.

What is the most likely diagnosis?

○ A Rheumatoid arthritis
○ B Dermatomyositis
○ C Systemic lupus erythematosus (SLE)
○ D Polyarthritis nodosa
○ E Henoch–Schönlein purpura

questions

218 A 2-week-old infant presents with a rash. Complications at birth included an irregular heartbeat and jaundice. On examination, you find a healthy male infant with a macular-papular discoid rash. He has a heart rate of 90 bpm with no murmurs and normal peripheral pulses. Gastrointestinal examination reveals a liver enlarged by 3 cm with a non-tender abdomen and normal bowel sounds. Investigations show an autoimmune haemolytic anaemia and thrombocytopenia. An ECG confirms bradycardia.

1   *Which of the following investigations will give a diagnosis in this baby?*

    ○ A Antinuclear antibody (ANA) antibody positive
    ○ B Rheumatoid factor positive
    ○ C Anti-double-stranded DNA negative
    ○ D Anti-Ro positive
    ○ E Anti-La positive

2   *Which of the following maternal results will shed light on the infant's diagnosis?*

    ○ A Anti-double-stranded DNA antibody
    ○ B Anti-cardiolipin antibody
    ○ C Anti-Ro antibody
    ○ D ANA antibody
    ○ E All of the above

3   *What is the likely diagnosis?*

    ○ A Drug-induced lupus
    ○ B Systemic lupus erythematosus (SLE)
    ○ C Neonatal lupus
    ○ D Lupus anticoagulant disorder
    ○ E Kasabach–Merritt's syndrome

Extended Matching Question

219 Theme: Vasculitides

A   Perinuclear antinuclear cytoplasmic antibody (ANCA) positive
B   Double-stranded DNA antibody positive
C   ANCA positive
D   Rheumatoid factor positive
E   Cytoplasmic ANCA positive
F   Antihistone antibody positive
G   Anticardiolipin antibody positive
H   Anti-rim antibody positive
I   Anti-Ro and anti-La antibody positive
J   Anti-single-stranded DNA antibody positive

Match the following three diseases with the appropriate results from investigations for vasculitides.

○   1   Polyarteritis nodosa
○   2   Microscopic polyangiitis
○   3   Wegener's granulomatosis

questions

Statistics

Question Frequency

Alternative hypothesis	1	Null hypothesis	1
Associations (adult)	3	Population (adult)	2
Bias	0	Prevalence	1
Case control study	1	Probability	3
Category frequency data	1	Randomisation	1
Clinical trials (adult)	4	Regression	0
Coefficient of variation	0	Reliability	0
Continuous data with normal		Sample distribution	3
distribution	0	Significance test	4
Correlation coefficient	3	Standard deviation	4
Data summary	0	Standard error (adult)	1
Degrees of freedom	0	Statistics	3
Diagnositc tests (adult)	6	t-test – unpaired	1
Experimental design	1	Trial	0
Incidents	1	Type of error	0
Measures of central tendency	1	Validity	0
Measures of variation	0		

questions

Multiple True/False Questions

220 The number-needed-to-treat (NNT) is

- ○ A The number of individuals who can come to harm from being treated
- ○ B Determined by the relative risk
- ○ C Worked out from the odds ratio
- ○ D Calculated by systematic review
- ○ E Derived from the absolute risk reduction

221 Which of the following are recognised types of bias?

- ○ A Selection
- ○ B Publication
- ○ C Recall
- ○ D Lost to follow-up
- ○ E Edgarian

222 Which of the following statements regarding confidence intervals is true?

- ○ A They tend to be larger the larger the sample size
- ○ B They give an idea of the range in which the true figure lies
- ○ C They are always quoted for the 5% and the 95% centiles
- ○ D They overlap in cases where the mean is higher than the mode
- ○ E They are derived from the odds ratio

223 In diagnostic testing, which of the following statements is correct?

- ○ A The test threshold is that below which treatment is not required
- ○ B The test threshold is always set at 25%
- ○ C The treatment threshold is the value above which treatment is not required
- ○ D The treatment threshold should be set at 85%
- ○ E The patient's clinical status should not have a bearing on the need for treatment

224 Of the following five statements regarding probability scores, which is correct?

- ○ A If $P = 0$, the outcome occurs
- ○ B If $P = 1$, the outcome never occurs
- ○ C If $P = 0.5$, the outcome will occur in 50% of cases
- ○ D 0.01 is more significant than 0.001
- ○ E 1% is more significant than 0.01%

questions

225 Of the following five formulae noted, which is the correct formula for standard error of the mean? N is the number of cases and SD is standard deviation.

○ A Standard error = variance/N
○ B Standard error is square root of N/SD
○ C Standard error is square root of SD/N
○ D Standard error is N/SD
○ E Standard error is SD/N

Best of Five Question

226 This correlation coefficient is used if one or both variables have a normal distribution. The correlation coefficient is used to determine whether there is a mathematical linear relationship between diastolic blood pressure and serum cholesterol levels in a group of patients with hypertension.

Of the following five coefficients, which is described?

○ A Parametric Pearson's correlation coefficient
○ B Non-parametric Spearman's correlation coefficient
○ C Kendall's rank correlation coefficient
○ D Chi-squared test
○ E Student's t-test

Extended Matching Questions

227 Theme: Diagnostic tests

A Sensitivity
B Specificity
C Positive predictive value
D Negative predictive value
E Precision
F Accuracy
G Incidence
H Prevalence
I Attack rate
J Mortality rate

Of the ten diagnostic tests, which is being described in the following three clinical scenarios?

○ 1 This is the proportion of true negatives that are correctly identified by a test and have true positives and a few false positives. It tells us about the false positives, and this category is good at excluding a disease. What is the diagnostic test?

○ 2 This category determines those which have a positive test and determines how many truly have the disease, ie are true positives and test positive. This depicts the chance that you may have the condition if your test result is positive.

○ 3 This is the number of new cases diagnosed per head of population in a given time, usually 1 year. A longitudinal study is used to determine this figure. What is this diagnostic statement?

228 Theme: Clinical trials

A Blind trial
B Single-blind trial
C Double-blind trial
D Triple-blind trial
E Double-blind placebo-controlled trial
F Parallel trial
G Crossover trial
H Controlled trial
I Randomisation
J Observational trial

Of the following ten clinical trials, which is discussed in each of the clinical scenarios?

○ 1 The patient and doctor are unaware of who receives the drug in question and who receives the placebo. What is the clinical trial?

○ 2 This trial occurs when each patient is exposed to both treatments, therefore allowing a comparison of each treatment. In the studies, a period of wash-out is essential to eradicate potential carry-over effects before commencing the second treatment. What is this clinical trial?

○ 3 This trial is conducted in a parallel fashion so each patient is exposed to only a single treatment. Multicentre designs are recommended to obtain sufficient cases. What is this clinical trial?

Vaccination

Question Frequency

BCG	0	Immunoglobulin	3
Bordetella pertussis	1	Inactivated live vaccines	3
Contraindications (adult)	2	Influenza	1
DPT	1	Killed vaccine	0
Haemophilus influenzae B	2	Measles	3
Hepatitis A	0	MMR	2
Hepatitis B	0	Polio	2
Immunisations	3	Polio oral Sabin	3

Multiple True/False Questions

229 Which of the following are true contraindications to pertussis immunisation?

- ○ A In a previous immunisation, inconsolable screaming for 72 hours
- ○ B A definite convulsion within 72 hours of a previous immunisation
- ○ C A progressive neurological condition
- ○ D Treatment with corticosteroids
- ○ E Treatment with antibiotics

230 Which of these statements are contraindications to the administration of live vaccines?

- ○ A Children with tuberculosis (TB) can be given measles vaccination only if they are not receiving TB treatment
- ○ B Live vaccine should not be given within 3 months after the child has received a normal dose of immunoglobulin
- ○ C Newly organ transplanted patients
- ○ D Jaundice in the neonatal period
- ○ E A family history of adverse reactions to immunisation

231 What type of vaccine is the Hib vaccine?

- ○ A Pertussal
- ○ B Acellular
- ○ C Conjugate/combined
- ○ D Virus extracted
- ○ E All of the above

232 Individuals should be given prophylactic Hib vaccine with which of the following diseases?

- ○ A Septic arthritis
- ○ B Sickle cell disease
- ○ C Periorbital cellulitis
- ○ D Asplenia
- ○ E Children who have had a splenectomy

Extended Matching Questions

233 Theme: Vaccination schedule

A DPT 3
B Polio 3
C Meningitis C 3
D Hib 3
E MMR
F BCG at birth
G Hepatitis B
H Rubella booster
I BCG
J DPT, meningitis C and polio booster

Match the vaccines above to the age group indicated as required under the UK immunisation scheme.

○ 1 10–14 years
○ 2 2, 3 and 4 months
○ 3 High-risk immigrants

234 Theme: Contraindications to vaccination

A Encephalitis
B High-dose corticosteroids
C An infant of, or a mother with, human immunodeficiency virus (HIV)
D Previous seizures
E A positive tuberculin test
F Immunocompromised host
G Pertussis infection
H Shock
I Disseminated BCGosis
J Atopy

Match the following three exclusion criteria to the ten clinical presentations.

○○○ 1 Which **three** of the above are contraindications for giving the DPT vaccine?

○○○○○ 2 Which **five** of the above are contraindications for giving a live vaccine?

○○ 3 Which **two** of the above are contraindications for giving the BCG vaccine?

235 Theme: Live and attenuated vaccines

A Polio (Salk)
B Cholera
C Yellow fever
D MMR
E Pneumococcal
F Polio (Sabin)
G Polysaccharide typhoid
H Live attenuated typhoid
I Hib
J Hepatitis B

Of the above vaccines routinely given to some children for prophylaxis:

   ○○○○ 1 Which **four** are live vaccines?

○○○○○○ 2 Which **six** are killed inactivated vaccines?

  ○○○○ 3 Which **four** are oral vaccines?

236 Theme: Identifying vaccines

A Varicella zoster immunoglobulin (ZIG)
B DPT
C Hepatitis B
D Measles
E BCG
F Rubella
G Polio (Salk)
H Polio (Sabin)
I Hib
J Pneumococcal

Match the following three descriptions of a vaccine to the list given above.

○ 1 A live vaccine given to males and females at 12–18 months of age irrespective of any previous history of viral infection. A booster may be given to girls at 12–14 years of age and within 72 hours of exposure to an infected contact. It has a high morbidity rate.

○ 2 A live vaccine containing an attenuated virus strain that is the most common cause of vaccine-related paralysis in the UK.

○ 3 A vaccine given to all children who are immunocompromised and who have recently been in contact with children with chicken pox or shingles.

Answers

Basic Science

Multiple True/False Answers

1 D

ANP was first discovered in 1981. It is a 21-amino-acid peptide. It is released from myocytes in response to an increase in atrial distension or stretch but NOT pressure. This may be due to volume overload such as occurs in congestive cardiac failure. It is secreted by both atria (right > left) and has a central role in volume homeostasis. It acts on the kidney to increase salt and water excretion and inhibit renin secretion. Three peptides have been discovered: A, B and C. Types B and C were both discovered in the brain, and type A and B receptors are active in signal transduction, whereas receptor C binds to peptides, thereby terminating their effect. The main functions of ANP in the kidney are:

- vasodilatation
- antagonism of the action of angiotensin II
- diminution of antidiuretic-hormone- (ADH-) induced water reabsorption in the collecting ducts
- inhibition of aldosterone, ADH and renin release, and an increase in sodium and water excretion
- reduction in blood pressure
- a negative effect on glomerular filtration rate
- a therapeutic role.

ANP may be used to treat hypertension, heart failure, myocardial infarction, cor pulmonale, left ventricular failure and ciclosporin toxicity. It is inactivated by neutral endopeptidases. These break down the natriuretic peptides and also other endogenous peptides such as bradykinin, substance P and angiotensin II.

answers

2 B

There is a stimulation of free nerve endings throughout both the left and right atria, and through myelinated and non-myelinated fibres in the vagus nerve. The efferent arc is activated via the sympathetic cardiac nerves. Activation of the arc causes:

- changes in renal blood flow
- changes in renal function
- changes in the tubule function of the demyelinated kidney.

The resulting stimulation of the atrial receptors causes an increase in water excretion and natriuresis in 5–10 minutes. The resulting physiological effects are:

- a decrease in antidiuretic hormone
- a decrease in renin
- a decrease in aldosterone.

Finally, peptides are excreted by the atria. Atrial natriuretic peptide inhibits sodium reabsorption in the distal nephron, causing the excretion of sodium and water but NOT potassium. Atrial natriuretic peptide antagonises the effects of noradrenaline and angiotensin II, especially in the context of vasoconstriction.

3 B

The technique of Southern blotting is named after Edward Southern. It is used to identify specific DNA fragments in a mixture of DNA.

The DNA to be analysed is digested with a restriction enzyme (endonuclease). The restricted fragments are separated according to size by gel electrophoresis. The separated fragments are then denatured by an alkali solution and transferred to a nitrocellulose or nylon filter by blotting. This process preserves the distribution of the fragments in the gel to produce a replica. This is absorbed on to the filter by capillary action.

A radiolabelled DNA probe is added and incubated with the restriction fragment. This probe may be P32, which sticks to the membrane. The DNA restriction fragment that is complementary to the probe hybridises with it and its location on the filter can be revealed by autoradiography. The configuration of the DNA isolated is then compared with that of the restriction map of cloned DNA.

This method is used to map restriction sites in genomic DNA next to a sequence of cloned DNA fragment. This allows a comparison of the restriction maps of different individual organisms in the region surrounding a cloned fragment. With this method, one is able to detect the deletion and insertion of mutations (if the noted mutation destroys or creates a restriction enzyme recognition site, it alters the size of the band on the exposed film) as well as sequencing differences in specific restriction sites.

Southern blotting has four main clinical applications:

1. In pre-natal diagnosis and counselling to determine mutations.
2. With infectious organisms to determine specific sequences for a given infection.
3. In tumour assessment to assess tumours for mutations in proto-oncogenes.
4. In forensic pathology to assess genomic imprinting.

4   A

Northern blotting demonstrates the presence or absence of specific whole RNA sequences in the tissues using a DNA probe.

The RNA sample is denatured with an agent that prevents hydrogen bonding between base pairs. This gives the RNA an unfolded configuration. The RNA is then separated on agarose gel via gel electrophoresis and transferred to a nitrocellulose or nylon filter, to which the denatured RNA adheres. This filter is then exposed to a labelled DNA probe and developed by autoradiography. This gives a semi-quantitative measure of RNA, allowing the amounts of particular mRNA in cells under different conditions to be compared.

5   C

Western blotting is used to detect a particular protein in a mixture. This process is also called immunoblotting (ELISA). There are four steps to this process:

Step 1: The protein mixture is separated on a polyacrylamide (SDS) gel.

Step 2: The face of the separated gel mixture is added to a nitrocellulose membrane, and the proteins bind. An electric field is applied that drives the proteins out of the gel and into the membrane.

Step 3: A (monoclonal) antibody specific to the protein of interest is added, and after incubation the membrane is washed to remove any unbound antibody. This is an alkaline phosphatase antibody that is linked and, when added, binds to the first antibody.

Step 4: Finally, a substrate is added and a purple precipitate is formed that marks the membrane band containing the protein of interest. The protein is thus identified.

answers

6 E

Cells that secrete antibody can be made immortal by fusing them with tumour cells and cloning the hybrids. Antibody secreted by hybridomas are specific for a single epitope on the variable Fab region of immunoglobulin. They are derived from a single B cell, and their specificity is of the parent type. These antibodies are made up of immortal clones and are therefore ideal partners for the fusion of B cells. In theory, unlimited quantities can be made.

Monoclonal antibodies are made by:

- the infusion of myeloma cells and B lymphocytes
- the immortalisation of B cells with Epstein–Barr virus
- the fact that they survive indefinitely and produce unlimited quantities of antibody.

The functions of monoclonal antibodies vary:

- Tumours have been targeted by attaching chemotherapeutic agents to monoclonal antibodies. They may therefore be used in the diagnosis of cancers and infections.
- They have been used as magic bullets to deliver drugs, pro-drugs and anti-toxins to a target.
- Their main use is in the diagnosis and research that is used to recognise a variety of cell markers.
- They are useful in medical imaging to image tumours and may assist in radiotherapy.
- They have been used in transplantation.

The side-effects are therefore those of any drug or anti-toxin, namely anaphylaxis.

Monoclonal antibodies may be used in various clinical contexts:

- *Monoclonal gammopathies*: These are a group of disorders associated with the production of monoclonal immunoglobulins or their constituents that are also known as plasma cell dyscrasias. These may include malignant myeloma, Waldenström's macroglobulinaemia and benign paraproteinaemia. They are the result of cellular dysregulation and NOT cell fusion. (Cell fusion in vitro results in hybridisation, which makes monoclonal antibody.) They may be made with IgG, IgA, IgM or IgD and hence some bind complement. They may produce IgG or IgM with rheumatoid factor activity (ie anti-idiotypes), although some symptoms may be attributable to hyperviscosity.
- *Waldenström's macroglobulinaemia*.
- *Cryoglobulinaemias*: IgM antibody may precipitate in the cold.

- *Myeloma – lytic bone lesions*: Myeloma is a malignant transformed B cell lineage that secretes a specific antibody. This fact is used to produce specific antibodies directed towards an antigen of choice. A laboratory animal is injected with an antigen of choice, an immune response is mounted, and the spleen is harvested. The cells fuse en masse to a specialised myeloma cell line that no longer produces its own cell body. The resulting fused cells – hybridomas – are immortal and produce antibody specified by lymphocytes to the immune animal. The cells can be screened to select for the antibody of interest, which can then be produced in limitless amounts.
- Excess light chains are produced in monoclonal gammopathies, but they are NOT all light chains as some may be whole immunoglobulins or heavy chains.

Best of Five Answers

7 C

Cancer, autoimmune and viral illnesses are associated with increased cell survival. For clinical use, apoptosis may be discussed in relation to various illnesses.

Malignancies. Metastatic tumour cells can survive in a foreign environment. The most common translocation in haematology is t(14:18), which is created by the *bcl-2* gene. Overexpression of bcl-2 specifically prevents cells from entering apoptosis, and expression has been correlated with poor survival from cancer. p53 protein is required for cells in which DNA has been damaged to undergo apoptosis. The failure of cells to die in a damaged environment may be due to the accumulation of the p53 gene mutation.

Viral illnesses. Death by apoptosis can be seen as an evolutionary adaptation to prevent the survival of virally infected cells. Viruses have found a method to avoid this. The pox virus inhibits apoptosis by producing an inhibitor of interleukin-1b-converting enzyme (ICE). Chicken pox does not appear to work in this way.

Degenerative disorders. The excessive cell death caused by excess cell signals may promote degenerative disorders.

Autoimmune diseases. Physiological death is necessary for the removal of potentially autoreactive T cells during development and for the removal of excess cells after the completion of the immune response. Animal models of SLE have implicated apoptosis in the pathogenesis of this autoimmune disease. An example is the loss of CD4 cells by apoptosis in AIDS.

Cells apoptose by five biochemical stages:

- shrinkage
- the condensation/cleavage of chromatin
- packaging of vesicles and marginalisation
- nuclear and cytoplasmic budding
- the formation of membrane-bound apoptotic bodies that are finally phagocytosed by macrophages.

8 C

TNF is present in the circulation in the free form and complexed to binding proteins derived from cleavage fragments of the TNF receptor. It has its receptors on nearly all nucleated cells except erythrocytes. It is produced from monocytes and macrophages, keratinocytes, renal cells, T, B and natural killer cells, as well as mast cells. These cells then release interferon-γ and cause changes in the endothelial cells. TNF promotes angiotensin and increases cell permeability and vascular leaking, promoting sites of inflammation. It also acts in a paracrine fashion at a site of release to promote inflammation/injury rather than repair or fibrosis.

TNF is not really used to target malignant cells. It is responsible for the severity of Gram-negative sepsis and is used to monitor the response to bacteria, viruses, other cytokines and immune complexes. It may induce granulocyte colony-stimulating factor and is an activator of monocytes and macrophages in diseased tissue. It is a co-stimulator for T cell activation and antibody production.

The cellular effects of TNF are:

- cytotoxicity to tumour cells and the promotion of tumour growth in culture
- the activation of inflammatory leukocytes to kill microbes
- the suppression of adipocyte lipoprotein lipase
- the reduction of myocyte resting membrane potential
- the stimulation of mononuclear phagocytes to produce cytokines
- an interferon effect against viruses
- co-stimulating the activation of T cells and antibody production via B cells.

The mechanisms of action of TNF are utilised in the pathology of many disorders and diseases.

Acute high exposure to TNF can occur in acute infections, when TNF contributes to the development of shock, pyrexia, vascular leak syndrome and widespread tissue injury. It is the principal mediator of the host response to Gram-negative bacteria and is therefore responsible for hypotension and hypercoagulability.

In chronic infections, there is chronic low exposure to TNF, causing cachexia, insulin resistance, hyperglycaemia, increased protein metabolism and anaphylaxis.

TNF is associated with malaria, rheumatoid arthritis and bone resorption. It gained its fame because anti-TNF antibody used to treat rheumatoid arthritis was so successful. In rheumatoid arthritis, it has a synergistic effect with interleukin-1 (IL-1). Both IL-1 and TNF are found on patients' synovial membranes. TNF-α has a strategy that induces monocytes to produce IL-1 at a level comparable to that of bacterial lipopolysaccharide. IL-1 can then activate osteoblasts and cause bone resorption, as well as activate fibroblasts to produce degradative enzymes.

Pathophysiology:

- TNF stimulates angiogenesis, which occurs with the inflammatory response.
- It is involved in the induction of apoptosis and necrosis, and thus regulates cell growth.
- It promotes the production of cytokines by mononuclear phagocytes.
- It is involved in the induction of leukocyte adhesion molecules (LAM and intra-cellular adhesion molecule (ICAM)).
- It upregulates leukocyte adhesion receptors on endothelial cells.
- It may be involved in the induction of necrosis of tumours (cytotoxicity).

TNF may be used in the treatment of malignant melanoma and other malignancies. An antibody to TNF is useful in rheumatoid arthritis but may not be helpful in shock.

Extended Matching Answer

9 Theme: Receptors

1 **E**

The TCR is a dimer and part of the CD3 complex. CD3 is closely related to the TCR and is responsible for communicating the antigen recognition signal into the cell, but it does not interact with it. The TCR is also an intracellular cell wall receptor like the steroid receptors. It detects antigen in association with HLA molecules via its immunoglobulin-like α and β or γ or δ chains. It works within the nuclear plasma membrane and the mitochondria.

The receptor is activated by antigen binding, which occurs by phosphorylation of the receptor and subsequent activation of the intracellular signal transduction pathway. Interleukin-2 release is increased by T cell activation, via its own receptor and NOT the TCR. The TCR interacts with processed antigen in the context of the histocompatibility complex I or II antigen depending on T cell type. The TCR does NOT interact with the CD3 complex, the class I complex or the β_2 microglobulin component per se.

2 **D**

The steroid receptor is part of the superantigen family. It has a similar action and structure to the thyroid and vitamin D receptors. It is located on the intracellular cell wall and works within the cytoplasmic environment. It is a nuclear hormone. When the chemical reacts with the ligand, it binds with *DNA* not RNA to cause an effect. This receptor is NOT blocked by aminoglutethimide, which inhibits the conversion of androgens to oestrogens in the tissues.

3 **F**

The LDL receptor is associated with abnormalities of chromosome 19. There are more than 100 mutations occurring in the genes encoding this receptor-mediated LDL catabolism, and these mutations can lead to the clinical syndrome of familial hypercholesterolaemia (autosomal dominant, F = M). The receptor is not restricted to the cell surface and continuously recycles from the cell surface to the endosomes (receptorsomes), internalising LDL for catabolism. High-density lipoprotein competes with LDL for receptor-mediated uptake.

Once internalised, LDL undergoes lysosomal degeneration, and its cholesterol ester is hydrolysed to free cholesterol. The release of this free cholesterol from the lysosome regulates cellular cholesterol content by:

- downregulating 3-hydroxy-3-methylglutaryl-CoA (HMG-CoA) reductase
- depressing LDL receptor synthesis
- activating acyl-CoA:cholesterol-*O*-acyltransferase (ACAT) so that any cholesterol surplus to requirement is converted to cholesterol ester and stored as droplets in the cytoplasm.

Cardiology

Multiple True/False Answers

10 ABE

ACE inhibitors are beneficial for both post-nephritic and renal hypertension but must be used with caution in patients with renal impairment. They are contraindicated for use in hypertension in pregnancy as they have teratogenic effects such as renal agenesis and hypoplasia, neonatal hypotension, cleft lip and palate deformities, and cardiac malformations. They must not be used to treat heart failure caused by aortic stenosis as there is an increased incidence of sudden death due to the precipitation of profound hypotension. Side-effects include cough, rash and angioneurotic oedema. Captopril and not enalapril causes dysquesia (loss or altered taste). ACE inhibitors do not cause gout or flushes.

Enalapril is used to treat hypertension and heart failure. It inactivates bradykinin in the conversion of angiotensin (AT) I to AT II in the lung epithelium. It therefore reduces the effects of AT II on aldosterone to cause hypotension in nephritic patients. It is a pro-drug that is converted to the active metabolite enalaprilat in the liver. It has a long half-life and is finally excreted via the kidneys. This metabolite is increased in the kidney in renal failure and therefore must be used with caution. Side-effects include hypotension, decreased renal function, neutropenia, angioneurotic oedema, non-productive cough and headaches but not flushing.

11 ACE

Chronic alcohol consumption results in dilated cardiomyopathy due to its toxic effects on the myocardium. Thiamine deficiency causes dilated cardiomyopathy as a result of a poor diet rather than directly because of the alcohol. Other cardiogenic effects include persistent chronic paroxysmal tachycardia and atrial fibrillation (not atrial flutter). There is a reported increased incidence of haemorrhagic and embolic stroke due to left atrial standstill, which may in turn precipitate the embolic phenomenon.

12 ABCE

Aortic valve stenosis is the aetiology underlying 5% of all cardiac malformations. It is more common in males than females, with a ratio of 3:1. It may be supravalvular, valvular or subvalvular, and there may be an association with a bicuspid aortic valve (as opposed to a tricuspid valve).

Clinically, the patient may be asymptomatic or present with symptoms and signs of aortic stenosis (AS) and aortic regurgitation (AR). There may be a palpable thrill in the suprasternal notch. There is an ejection systolic murmur at the upper right second intercostal space that radiates to the external carotid. At the apex, there are a diastolic murmur and an ejection click. The second heart sound may be soft. Hypotension is a feature. In severe circumstances, patients may present with chest pain, dizziness or palpitations on exertion, congestive cardiac failure, sudden collapse, arrhythmia, loss of consciousness or SIDS. There are no central nervous system sequelae. Exercise strategies are limited.

The ECG may be normal, but in severe cases left ventricular hypertrophy is seen with sinus rhythm (SR), a normal axis and LVS strain with ST depression and T wave inversion (especially on exercise). The chest radiograph may show enlargement of the left ventricle.

Treatment includes balloon valvuloplasty, balloon dilatation and valve replacement. Complications after repair include a mediastinotomy scar, a residual murmur of AS/AR and re-stenosis.

Associations include Williams' syndrome (supravalvular), Turner's syndrome, fetal phenytoin syndrome, coarctation of the aorta, hypertrophic obstructive cardiomyopathy (HOCM), hypoplastic left ventricle and mitral valve abnormality.

Supravalvular aortic stenosis is associated with diffuse or localised narrowing above the aortic sinus and the coronary arteries. It may be caused by peripheral pulmonary artery stenosis (PPAS) or peripheral branch arterial stenosis (PBAS) and may present similarly to AS. A differential diagnosis includes aortic stenosis (AS) and HOCM. Supravalvular aortic stenosis is classically associated with Williams' syndrome: dysmorphic facies, round face, full cheeks and lips, stellate iris, strabismus, learning difficulties, SVAO and hypercalcaemia.

Subaortic stenosis shows a fibrous diaphragm below the aortic valve. The region below the aorta is abnormal in most cases. It is often seen in conjunction with coarctation of the aorta. The clinical signs are similar to AS, but there is no EC. Surgery includes excision of the fibrous diaphragm. There is a strong relationship with bacterial endocarditis so prophylaxis is considered if the valve remains abnormal.

13 A

ASDs present in 8–10% of all cases of congenital heart disease. They present as acyanotic left-to-right shunts and are more common in the female population. ASDs can be divided into three types:

Ostium secundum (70%) fossa ovalis. This may be asymptomatic and is seen with a high incidence of sinus node disease. It may present with pulmonary hypertension (increasing shunt size), right ventricular failure in the third or fourth decade of life (NOT in infancy), and atrial arrythmias in adults with atrial fibrillation, flutter and tachycardia (rarely in childhood). ASDs are well tolerated in pregnancy unless there is pulmonary hypertension (PHT). ECG changes include right axis deviation, right ventricular hypertrophy, rSR, rsR, a prolonged PR interval and right bundle branch block. Right ventricular heave, a split second sound, a pansystolic murmur and a tricuspid diastolic murmur are all common clinical presentations. Surgery is beneficial if the pulmonary:systemic ratio is greater than 2:1 (left:right). A high peripheral pulmonary vascular resistance (PPVR) is a contraindication to surgery. NO antibiotic prophylaxis is required as the velocity gradient is low.

Ostium primum (30%). These defects lie close to the atrioventricular valve and the inter-atrial septum, and may therefore present earlier. They are often associated with an abnormality of the atrioventricular valve, a ventricular septal defect (VSD) or a complete atrioventricular septal defect. They may be associated with tricuspid regurgitation (TR) or mitral regurgitation (MR). ECG changes include left axis deviation, a prolonged PR interval and right bundle branch block. These defects DO require prophylactic antibiotics.

Sinus venosus (10%). These defects are situated high in the septum near the superior vena cava. They are frequently associated with total anomalous pulmonary venous drainage. Clinically, there is a left parasternal heave but no thrill, and wide fixed splitting of the second heart sound due to an increased PVR. The pansystolic murmur at the upper left sternal edge (ULSE) is due to flow across the pulmonary and a mid-diastolic tricuspid flow murmur. The sounds are therefore NOT due to the ASD defect. A large murmur at the LLSE indicates a large left-to-right shunt. The classic pulmonary systolic murmur lessens and disappears as pulmonary hypertension (PHT) develops.

Associations include Down's syndrome, asplenia, polysplenia, endocarditis and sick sinus syndrome. Complications include MR, TR and PHT (increased flow left-to-right shunt), and in childhood a common presentation is heart failure. Adults can present in the third decade of life with atrial arrythmias, PHT and heart failure.

answers

Investigations such as transoesophageal echography and a chest radiograph are required. The chest radiograph shows pulmonary plethora and increased blood flow.

Fewer than 10% of defects close spontaneously; primary lesions often present in adulthood and are usually symptomatic and need surgery. All secondary lesions must be closed in childhood. Spontaneous closure is, as for VSD, is uncommon. Antibiotic prophylaxis must be given in adults.

14 ABCE

Atrial fibrillation is seen in ischaemic heart disease, thyrotoxicosis, mitral valve disease, sick sinus syndrome, myocarditis, cardiomyopathy, constrictive pericarditis, ASD in adults but not children, pulmonary embolism and cancer of the bronchus.

Atrial fibrillation occurs when the heart rate is 400–700 bpm; the ventricular rate is irregular with fibrillatory waves. There are NO P waves. In atrial flutter, the rate is 200–400 bpm and the rate is regular. Flutter gives a sawtooth appearance on ECG. Fibrillation is rare in childhood and is seen usually when there are structural defects, surgery to the atria, ie after an ASD repair, myocardial disease or Wolff–Parkinson–White syndrome (the complexes are broad).

Treatment includes DC external cardioversion, rapid digitalisation or digoxin (avoid in Wolff–Parkinson–White as it facilitates conduction down the incorrect pathway – use flecainide, amiodarone or disopyramide instead). Other drugs to use are disopyramide and amiodarone. Anticoagulation must be used in chronic heart failure prior to conversion to prevent atrial thrombi causing an embolism. This stage gives a poor prognosis.

Paroxysmal atrial tachycardia presents with a heart rate of over 150 bpm and causes syncope and an abrupt decrease in heart rate in response to carotid massage. It terminates re-entry by increasing atrioventricular block and decreasing ventricular rate. It can cause asystole, and it compromises cardiac output. It does not cause pulsus paradoxus.

15 ABCE

Atrial flutter is rare and occurs when there is a re-entry loop within the atrium. There is atrioventricular (AV) block with typically 2:1 conduction. The heart rate is 250–350 bpm, with an average of 300 bpm. The atrial rate is 100 bpm. The ECG shows a sawtooth pattern. The degree of AV block can be increased by vagal stimulation, in which the ventricular rate is suddenly slowed and there is an increase in atrial flutter; this may be diagnostic. When the heart rate increases, the AV node is unable to respond, leading to AV block. There is a regular ventricular rate of 2:1, 3:1,

4:1 or 3:2 (Wenkebach's phenomenon), becoming irregular if this pattern varies. Therefore, regular and irregular are both correct!

Clinically, there is a regular/irregular pulse, cardiac pain or syncope. It may be treated with quinidine, which slows the flutter rate and increases AV conduction. Digitalis may be needed as well. Carotid massage will decrease the ventricular rate, and sinus rhythm may be restored by DC shock cardioversion. If it is intractable, use verapamil or a β blocker.

Organic disease of the heart may be present, for example myocardial infarction and angina pectoris. It can occur after cardiac surgery, acute infection, endocarditis and myocarditis.

Best of Five Answers

16 D

Coarctation of the aorta occurs in 4% of all congenital heart disease. It is more prominent in males than females and is associated with trisomy 13 and 18, Turner's syndrome, valproate toxicity and abnormalities of ventricular septal defect, persistent ductus arteriosus, mitral valve abnormalities and berry aneurysms of the circle of Willis. Other associated cardiac abnormalities include bicuspid aortic valve (70%), mitral valve disease, aortic regurgitation (20%) and subaortic stenosis. Ninety-eight per cent of coarctations occur at the level of the pulmonary artery after the subclavian artery. It is for this reason that, on observation, the proximal blood pressure varies compared with the distal blood pressure. The blood pressure in the right arm is often greater than that in the left arm. Clinically, these children present with hypertension, prominent carotid pulses, radiofemoral delay, left ventricular hypertrophy and an ejection systolic murmur maximum over the posterior left interscapular area. An apical click over the aortic valve may be heard. Coarctation of the aorta may be simple (post-ductal) or complex (pre-ductal or with a septal defect), and may be associated with aortic stenosis, transposition of the great arteries or a bicuspid aortic valve.

The ECG and chest radiograph may be normal. However, as the child enters the first decade, evidence of cardiomegaly, congestive heart failure, post-stenotic dilatation with a dilated subclavian artery and rib notching may be noticed. The ECG may show right ventricular hypertrophy, left ventricular hypertrophy in infancy and right axis deviation. Complications of coarctation of the aorta include left ventricular failure, cerebral haemorrhage, aortic dissection, renal vascular stenosis and infective endocarditis. This condition may result in death due to an aortic aneurysm

answers

or rupture in the third or fourth decade of life. It may also cause premature ischaemic heart disease as a result of hypertension. If left untreated, 20% of individuals die before 20 years of age and 80% before 50 years of age. Treatment options include surgical balloon dilatation or the grafting of a subclavian flap, and should surgical correction not normalise the blood pressure, further medical management is required.

17 E

Rheumatic fever occurs because of an abnormal immune response to a streptococcal antigenetic component. It has a latent period of 1–3 weeks and is more common in the lower socio-economic classes. It peaks at around 5–15 years of age and affects the blood vessels, joints, nervous system and subcutaneous tissues. It is characterised as an autoimmune disease, and there is a risk of rheumatic fever occurring after infection in 3% of the population. The recurrence is greater in younger children and increases with each attack. Rheumatic fever is categorised according to the Duckett-Jones criteria, which are as follows:

- *Major:* carditis 50%, chorea (Sydenham's) 15%, polyarthritis (flitting) 70%, erythema marginatum 10%, subcutaneous nodules (painless) 1%.
- *Minor:* arthralgia, fever, prolonged PR interval, raised ESR, raised CRP.

Supporting evidence is a previous history of rheumatic fever, evidence of streptococcal disease from a throat swab, a raised ASO titre and a positive streptococcal antigen test or a leukocytosis.

In order to make the diagnosis of rheumatic fever, two major and/or one major with two minor criteria are required. Evidence of a recent streptococcal infection with a raised ASO titre or an antiribonuclease B level is sufficient. Exceptions are as follows:

- chorea alone is diagnostic
- an insidious or late-onset carditis with no other explanation
- rheumatic recurrence, one major and one minor criterion with prior streptococcal disease that is recurring.

Consequences of pericarditis include heart block, pericardial effusion, tachycardia, cardiomegaly, pericardial friction rub, congestive cardiac failure, valvular disease and a Carey–Coombes apical mid-diastolic rumbling murmur. New heart murmurs are often audible, including those of mitral regurgitation and aortic regurgitation. Skin nodules affect the perivascular tissues and are non-specific lesions resulting from fibroid degeneration. Medication includes aspirin for the acute phase, non-steroidal anti-inflammatory drugs for the arthritis, prednisolone for severe carditis, and high-dose penicillin for immediate management with antibiotic prophylaxis in the long term. Antibiotics may include penicillin V, erythromycin or benzyl penicillin. Diazepam and haloperidol may be required to control the chorea.

answers

18 B

WPWS has an incidence of 1.5/1000 cases and is more common in boys and men. The most common presentation is with re-entry tachycardia due to an aberrant re-entry circuit at the bundle of Kent. WPWS displays an atrial ventricular re-entry tachycardia that may be regular or irregular. This abnormality shows a disorder of the pathway between the atrial and ventricular myocardium, and it may present with superventricular tachycardia owing to pre-excitation; it therefore presents in regular arrhythmia as a recurrent supraventricular tachycardia but not a ventricular tachycardia in 10%. It may be due to an anomalous atrial ventricular conduction pathway.

WPWS is associated with mitral valve prolapse, commonly seen in Marfan's syndrome, corrected transposition of the great arteries, Epstein's anomaly (as in this case) and atrial septal defect (ostium secundum). It is also found in hypertrophic obstructive cardiomyopathy, but it is not associated with myocarditis, tamponade or a vein of Galen abnormality. In the adult population, it may be associated with thyrotoxicosis and lithium ingestion during the antenatal period. In this case, Epstein's anomaly is associated with displacement of the septal and posterior leaflets of the tricuspid valve. This causes atrialisation of part of the right ventricle and subsequent cyanosis and heart failure.

WPWS is usually diagnosed on the ECG, which shows a short PR interval, a widened QRS complex and a delta wave. There is a dominant R in V1 with left-sided right bundle branch block pattern in type A WPWS, whereas in type B there is a left bundle branch block pattern that is right-sided with no dominant R wave in V1. There may be associated inverted T waves in the anterior leads. In the older population, WPWS presents most commonly with atrial ventricular re-entry tachycardia, which shows regular narrow complex arrhythmia in 70% of cases. However, 10–15% may present in atrial fibrillation and 5% in atrial flutter, and it is rare to have atrial ventricular non-re-entry circuit tachycardia.

Clinically, infants present in heart failure. The older population may present with dizziness, dyspnoea and palpitations. Prophylaxis may be controlled with class 1C verapamil, and surgical intervention includes radiofrequency ablation, which has a 90% cure rate. Amiodarone may be highly effective for all arrhythmias in the refractory period to prevent development of the accessory pathway but should be avoided in the blocked atrial ventricular node. Long-term use can lead to thyroid problems. Flecainide is also successful for dysrhythmias; it is, however, not used in adults. In infants, it is good maintenance therapy. Long-term verapamil treatment may cause hypotension, and sotalol is avoided in the under-12-month age group, as is digoxin.

Clinical Pharmacology

Multiple True/False Answers

19 D

Glucocorticoids include cortisone and hydrocortisone, which have a low mineralocorticoid activity, along with prednisolone, betamethasone and dexamethasone. For replacement therapy, hydrocortisone in combination with fludrocortisone is used; this latter drug has little anti-inflammatory activity.

The strength of the anti-inflammatory effects of 5 mg prednisolone =

- Betamethasone 750 μg
- Cortisone acetate 25 mg
- Deflazacort 6 mg
- Dexamethasone 750 μg
- Hydrocortisone 20 mg
- Methylprednisolone 4 mg.

20 CDE

Antacids tend to alkalinise the urine, leading to increased urinary aspirin clearance, whereas metoclopramide enhances its absorption. Aspirin diminishes the actions of uricosuric agents such as probenicid and sulfinpyrazone.

21 DE

The following are first-line treatments for the other conditions:

- rheumatic fever: phenyloxymethylpenicillin
- meningococcal meningitis: rifampicin (ciprofloxacin for pregnant women and young children)
- *Haemophilus influenzae* type B: rifampicin.

22 ABCDE

Repeated doses may be required. Giving the activated charcoal with a small quantity of squash and using a straw may make it more palatable.

23 ABC

The main effects of pethidine can be reversed by naxolone, the liver damage associated with paracetamol overdose can be reduced/eliminated with the use of N-acetyl cysteine, and chelating agents can be used with iron poisoning.

24 E

NSAIDs are disease-modifying drugs. They decrease the antihypertensive effect of angiotensin-converting enzyme inhibitors and therefore increase the risk of renal failure and hyperkalaemia. They antagonise the effects of β-blockers and inhibit cyclo-oxygenase.

Many of the renal side-effects arise from the prostaglandin-inhibiting properties of NSAIDs. In the kidney NSAIDs cause vasoconstriction, a decreased glomerular filtration rate and sodium and water retention, oppose the action of loop diuretics, augment the action of antidiuretic hormone (water retention) and cause hypernatraemia, hyperaldosteronism and hyperkalaemia. Side-effects of using NSAIDs include interstitial nephritis and nephrotic proteinuria but not nephrotic syndrome. Eosinophilic infiltrates are often found on biopsy. Other complications include nausea and rashes.

Best of Five Answers

25 B

Amiodarone has the above properties, successfully suppresses an arrhythmia and does not cause mortality. It was used in the Basal Anti-arrhythmic Study of Infarction Survey (BASIS) and found to be of benefit. It decreased all arrhythmias compared with a placebo and other antiarrhythmic medication. The study did, however, conclude that β-blockers were still the best medication for a post-myocardial infarct.

Amiodarone potentiates digoxin, as it competes with it at digoxin-binding sites, warfarin, other antiarrhythmics and iodine content. It may therefore potentiate hyperthyroidism and may subsequently inhibit the conversion of thyroxine to active T_3 and cause hypothyroidism. Other side-effects include reversible corneal microdeposits, optic neuritis, slate-grey skin syndrome, photosensitivity, pulmonary fibrosis, alveolitis, hepatitis, peripheral neuropathy, myopathy, hyperthyroidism, hypothyroidism (10%), heart block, dermatitis, tremor, gastrointestinal disturbance, lung amiodarone pulmonary disease, bradycardia, raised intracranial pressure, vasculitis and thrombocytopenia. It may be well tolerated in low doses and is effective in the prevention and cardioversion of atrial flutter and fibrillation.

answers

26 A

Sodium valproate has many dose-related side effects, including thrombocytopenia, tremor, appetite stimulation, alopecia, ataxia, fatal hepatitis, gastric irritation, pancreatitis, menstrual irregularities, encephalopathy, hyperammonaemia (20%) and hepatotoxicity (1 in 20 000). Plasma levels are required to determine the efficacy of the clinical response. Sodium valproate is not used for infantile spasms (nitrazepam, adrenocorticotrophic hormone or prednisolone are used instead) or status epilepticus (lorazepam and phenytoin).

27 C

This girl has presented in a compensated metabolic acidosis due to the accumulation of organic acid secondary to salicylate poisoning. All her symptoms are those found in the acute phase of the condition, and loss of consciousness is found in the late phase. Other presenting features and complications include hyperventilation, hyperpyrexia, dehydration, pulmonary oedema, acute renal failure and irritability.

Physiologically, as there is an increase in initial respiratory alkalosis, bicarbonate is released in the urine, causing hyponatraemia and hypokalaemia, and water is released in the urine. This therefore causes a compensatory metabolic acidosis, promoting the accumulation of lactate pyruvate. A stimulation of fat catabolism leads to ketone and β-hydroxybutyrate production, an increase in protein catabolism and aminoaciduria.

Treatment includes emesis and gastric lavage with activated charcoal. Electrolytes and renal function need to be corrected, and a forced alkaline diuresis with 0.9% saline, 5% dextrose and 1.26% bicarbonate solution is required to keep the pH of the urine between 7.5 and 8.5. The initial hyperventilation in the acute phase causes the respiratory alkalosis and thus the compensatory metabolic acidosis, which in turn causes the ketonuria. With regard to the significance of the serum dose levels at 6 hours, the following should be remembered:

- 3–500 mg/l is mild
- 500–750 mg/l is moderate
- >750 mg/l is severe.

Dermatology

Best of Five Answers

28 D

Incontinentia pigmenti is a multisystem disorder that shows dominant inheritance. It affects only girls and women clinically as the condition is lethal in males in utero. If a diagnosis is difficult, a look at the mother is always suggested. Clinically there are three phases: (1) the bullous phase – crops of vesicles appear in the first 2 weeks of life; (2) the papular phase – warty papules that flatten out over the skin; and (3) the hyperpigmented phase – pigmentary changes in the form of whorls and streaks that are hypo- and hyperpigmented in nature. There is a different level of melanosis present in each whorl. As this is a multisystem disorder, other clinical symptoms and signs include dental and ocular anomalies, seizures in 30% of cases, rarely learning difficulties, although some children will have a decreased IQ, musculoskeletal abnormalities, alopecia and wiry hair.

On skin biopsy, there will be a marble-like lesion that runs in a linear streak, and the skin may appear blistered with a normal or decreased number of melanocytes and hyperkeratosis. There are a large number of intradermal eosinophils but no inflammatory cells. As the child grows older, there will be residual hyperpigmented whorls. The lesions appear in early childhood and then leave a grey streaky pigmentation in adulthood. The differential diagnosis is as in the question.

29 C

There are three main types of tinea infection, which are very difficult to distinguish clinically but have different aetiological factors.

- Tinea versicolor. The fungus responsible for this infection is *Pityrosporum orbiculare* (*Malassezia furfur*). On dark skin, multiple hypopigmented macules with a scaly component are visible. On fair skin, hyperpigmented lesions can be seen. This is not vitiligo, which has a convex edge to it and when investigated has an associated autoimmune component.

answers

- Tinea capitis. This skin disease is caused by *Trichophyton*.
- Tinea corporis. This is commonly known as ringworm and is caused by a dermatophyte infection *Microsporum canis*. The lesions appear to be annular and erythematous with a scaly, pruritic border and a clear centre. The diagnosis is made by skin scrapings. Treatment is antifungal medication for the skin, hair and nails.

Extended Matching Answers

30 Theme: Rashes

1 **C**

Erythema multiforme is a self-limiting and recurring condition that affects the skin and mucosal surfaces. The disease involves inflammatory eruptions characterised by symmetrical erythematous, oedematous or bulbous lesions of the skin and mucosal membranes. They look like target lesions with a purple or pale centre surrounded by red rings from macules that then form blisters. Involvement of the mucosal membranes includes debilitating stomatitis and conjunctivitis. Children may suffer from a persistent fever, malaise, photophobia and arthralgia.

Causes of erythema multiforme are multiple, but important ones to consider include herpes simplex virus, *Mycoplasma* and orf virus. Bacterial causes include *Streptococcus*, *Yersinia enterocolitica*, *Mycobacterium tuberculosis* and *Salmonella typhi/paratyphi*. Systemic lupus erythematosus, polyarteritis nodosa and collagen vascular diseases are all autoimmune disorders. Histoplasmosis, carcinoma, lymphomas and leukaemias may be associated oncological factors. Important drugs to consider include sulphonamide, penicillin, barbiturate, sulphonylurea, salicylate, phenytoin, L-dopa and chlorpropamide.

2 **D**

There are two clinical alternatives that may present as erythema multiforme. There is mild erythema multiforme that presents with symmetrical target lesions that are non-pruritic and may be bulbous in nature and resolve after 4–6 weeks. Severe erythema multiforme may, however, present as Stevens–Johnson syndrome whereby a severe erythema multiforme rash appears with bullae of the mouth, anogenital region and conjunctivae. Death occurs in 5–20% of cases. Systemic effects include polyarthritis, pneumonia and severe fluid and electrolyte imbalance. Treatment options include mouthwashes, antibiotics to treat secondary infection, steroids, ophthalmic care and intensive care support.

3 **A**

Chronic idiopathic urticaria is always part of the differential diagnosis for the above two clinical scenarios.

Development

Multiple True/False Answers

31 C

The following gives a rough estimation of a child's drawing skills from the drawing category of the Ruth Griffiths mental developmental scales, established from the modified Benet and Bender Gestalt test. Children are asked to draw independently a straight line, a horizontal line, a circle, a cross, a square or a man. The ages at which these are *copied* and *not imitated* are established as follows:

1 Can hold a pencil as if to mark a paper – 11 months

   Uses pencil on paper a little – 13 months

   Scribbles – 18–28 months

   Circular scribble in imitation – 2.5–3 years

   Perpendicular stroke or line in imitation – 2 years

2 Perpendicular stroke without imitation – 3 years

   Horizontal line – 3 years

   Copies a circle or a cross – 3 years

3 Copies a ladder, stage I – 4 years

   Draws a man, stage I – 4 years

4 Copies a square – 5 years

   Draws a primitive house with windows, stage I – 5 years

5 Draws a man, stage II – 6 years

   Triangle – 6 years

   Three letters – 6 years

   Writes or prints first name – 6 years

   Draws a house, stage II – 6 years

Draws a slanted rectangle – 6 years

Draws a precise ladder, stage II – 6 years

6 Draws a diamond – 7 years

Writes figures to 9 correctly – 7 years

Writes his or her full name – 7 years

7 Draws a blocked cross and circle/diamond touching – 8 years

Writes 10+ letters – 8 years

Draws a man, stage II – 8 years

8 Draws a tube – 9 years

32 E

The assessment of children's hearing can often be difficult and inconclusive. A significant family history must be sought and any parental doubt of a child's hearing investigated. Hearing assessment includes both a parental questionnaire and a clinical assessment. A hearing deficit is usually suspected if there is an articulation defect at 6.5 months of age. Developmental milestones of hearing are shown in Table 1.

Milestone	Age (months)
Turn to sound	3–6
Hearing on a horizontal plane	6
Hearing below a horizontal plane	7
Hearing above a horizontal plane	8

Table 1: Milestones in hearing

Hearing assessment tests vary for different ages of children in order to adapt to their level of cooperation (Table 2).

Test	Notes	Age
Startle test	Freezes to bell 8–13 cm away	6 weeks
Distraction test	Two assessors	7–15 months
Toy test	Kendall and McCormack	2 years
Pure tone audiometry	Pictures with conditioned responses and a Stycar chart	3 years
Picture test	Six pictures and 12 pictures	3 years for 6 pictures 4 years for 12 pictures

Table 2: Hearing assessment tests

answers

answers

Other tests include auditory response cradles, oto-acoustic emissions, brainstem-evoked auditory responses. A rough age guideline is shown in Table 3.

Age	Tests used
0–6 months	Objective, brainstem-evoked auditory responses, oto-acoustic emission
6–18 months	Distraction tests
6–24 months	Visual reinforcement audiometry
18–24 months	Cooperation tests, play audiometry
2–3 years	Sound field conditioning (headphones)
3–6 years	Pure tone audiometry

Table 3: Age guidelines for hearing tests

33 D

Head lag and a tonic neck reflex posture with the head to one side are seen up to 6 weeks of age for a full-term infant. Crawling is attempted at 7–8 months of life, and sitting with support is achieved by 5–6 months.

34 ABCH

E is attained at 3 years, D and F at 4 years and G at 5 years. H is a skill that is possible from 15–18 months of age onwards.

35 AB

At 3 months of age, the child reacts to sudden noises, quietens or stills to the mother's or father's voice, vocalises in a happy manner when spoken to, cries when uncomfortable or irritated, and stills to a bell or rattle for 3–5 seconds.

At 12 months, the child is eagerly attentive to sounds, vocalises deliberately as a means of communication, being either friendly or annoyed, shouts for attention, babbles considerably, understands 'no' and 'bye bye', and imitates adults engaging in playful sounds.

36 None is correct

At 18 months, the following gross motors skills would be expected:

- walks with the feet slightly apart
- runs carefully with the head held high
- pushes and pulls objects around the floor
- walks upstairs if the hand is held
- kneels on a flat surface without support.

At 2 years, the following would be seen:

- squats to play with toys and can rise to the feet without using the hands
- climbs on to furniture and can get down again
- walks upstairs holding on to a rail or the wall, with two feet on each step
- throws a ball overhand forwards without falling over
- sits on a small tricycle and propels forwards by pushing with the feet on the floor

At 2.5 years of age, these would be the normal gross milestones to have been achieved:

- walks upstairs confidently
- runs in straight lines
- can jump with two feet together from the lowest step
- can stand on tiptoe
- should be able to cast a hand-held ball somewhat stiffly at body level.

Best of Five Answers

37 C

Pendred's syndrome is the most common form of inherited congenital deafness. It is inherited in an autosomal recessive fashion and presents with a simple euthyroid goitre and mild hypothyroidism. The congenital deafness is usually sensorineural in nature. Other genetic disorders associated with hearing loss include Down's syndrome, velocardiofacial syndrome, Treacher Collins syndrome, Goldenhaar syndrome, Alport's syndrome, CHARGE syndrome and heterochromia. Waardenburg's syndrome is a rare autosomal dominant disorder, the deafness being associated with pigmentary anomalies including a white forelock, heterochromia iridis and facial abnormalities.

Acquired causes for hearing loss include chronic suppurative otitis media, commonly known as glue ear. This is the most common cause of deafness and speech delay in children, causes including allergy, rhinitis, hay fever, malformation of the eustachian tube and the accumulation of fluid in the middle ear. Other infective causes include otitis media, meningitis secondary to a *Pneumococcus* or *Haemophilus influenzae* infection and encephalitis secondary to mumps or *Haemophilus influenzae*, but not toxoplasmosis, as this presents with choroidoretinitis.

38 C

The primitive reflexes are indicators of functional integrity and maturity. The majority of reflexes do not persist beyond 6 months of age. There are 13 reflexes of importance, including:

- Moro reflex
- startle reflex
- rooting reflex
- sucking reflex
- grasp reflex
- voluntary palmar grasp reflex
- voluntary reach reflex
- stepping reflex
- asymmetrical tonic clonic (crossed adductor) reflex
- parachute reflex
- Babinski plantar reflex
- tendon reflex
- clonus.

Note that gastrocolic reflux is not a primitive reflex.

Ninety-five per cent of reflexes will have disappeared by the ages shown in Table 4.

Age	Reflex lost
4 months	Palmar, placing, rooting reflexes
6 months	Primary parachute, Moro, crossed adductor, tonic clonic reflexes
9 months	Plantar reflexes

Table 4: Disappearance of reflexes

Extended Matching Answers

39 Theme: Developmental regression

1 **B – Batten disease**

2 **G – Subacute sclerosing panencephalopathy**

3 **J – Hydrocephalus secondary to a medulloblastoma**

The ten diagnoses are possible causes for a child presenting with developmental regression. Mitochondrial disorders include Leigh's encephalopathy and Batten disease. Batten disease often presents with myoclonic jerks, dementia and optic atrophy, with lipofuscin found in the bone marrow cells.

Lysosomal enzyme disorders include mucopolysaccharidoses, sphyngolipidoses (Gaucher's disease) and glycogen protein degradation disorders. These children present with abnormal facies, with or without hepatosplenomegaly. Other lysosomal enzyme disorders include mucolipidosis, Niemann–Pick disease (sphyngomyelin and cholesterol in the tissues, and foam cells present in bone marrow), and finally metachromic leukodystrophy, which includes neuropsychoses with associated hyporeflexia and peripheral neuropathy.

Neurocutaneous disorders include neurofibromatosis and tuberous sclerosis. Metabolic disorders include aminoacidurias, and infective causes such as herpes encephalopathy. Spieler–Mayer–Schrögen syndrome is associated with decreased visual acuity, seizures, developmental deterioration, spasticity, dystonia and akinesia.

The above disorders may be a cause of a child presenting with developmental regression at less than 3 years of age. Children presenting at over 3 years of age may have subacute sclerosing panencephalopathy secondary to measles, mitochondrial disorders as above, or genetic disorders of the grey and white matter.

40 Theme: Speech delay

1   **G – Emotional deprivation**

2   **C – Secretory otitis media**

3   **E – Autism**

In order to understand speech delay, the speech milestones in Table 5 should be understood

Age	Achievement
3–6 months	Tuneful vocalisations
6–12 months	Babble and repetitive syllables
	Mama, dada by 18 months said appropriately, by 12–14 months inappropriately
1–1.5 years	Words understood in opposite context with a good understanding of language
1.5–2.5 years	Jargon and intelligible words. By 2 years, may join two or more words together; asks why? and where?
2.5–4 years	Rapid speech development. Asks questions and may now direct speech to others
4+ years	May narrate stories. Is able to use grammar and sentences by 4.5 years

Table 5: Speech milestones

Causes of speech delay are many. Emotional deprivation is not an emotional disorder. It may be constitutional and is due to understimulation and neglect. It often occurs in single-child families or in families with multiple siblings where the youngest child is obviously neglected or spoken for by the elder siblings. It is not found in twins as they often speak to each other. Hearing deficit may be a cause of speech delay; causes include secretory otitis media and deafness. Communication disorders are often associated with speech and language delay; this may include autistic spectrum disorder, elective mutism and bilingual children. Other important causes of speech and language delay are listed in Table 6.

Condition	
Syndromes	Tuberous sclerosis
	Down's syndrome
	Fragile X syndrome
	Fetal alcohol syndrome
Neurological conditions	Cerebral palsy
	West's syndrome
	Duchenne muscular dystrophy
Metabolic disorders	Phenylketonuria
	Hypothyroidism
Infections	Intrauterine infections (TORCH)
	Meningitis

Table 6: Causes of speech and language delay

Differential diagnoses that affect but do not delay speech include tongue-tie, cleft palate and malocclusion. Cystinuria does *not* cause speech delay.

Embryology

Multiple True/False Answers

41 A

In the first week of life in utero (1/40), the embryo derives its nutrients and discards its waste by a simple process of diffusion. Development of the uteroplacental circulation commences at 9 days and is fully established within the third week after fertilisation (3/40). The cytotrophoblast proliferates, and processes form the primary stem villi. Further differentiation of the mesoderm forms the blood vessels, which subsequently connect with the vessels forming in the embryo. These differentiated structures are called the tertiary stem villi. Gases, nutrients and wastes diffuse between maternal and fetal blood between four established layers: (1) the endothelium of the villus capillaries; (2) the villus connective tissue; (3) a layer of cytotrophoblast; and (4) a layer of syncytiotrophoblast. The placenta contains 150 ml of maternal blood and is replaced 3–4 times per minute. Carbon dioxide, urea and uric acid pass from the fetal to the maternal blood as waste.

42 C

The pharyngeal pouches consist of bars of mesenchymal tissue separated from each other by pharyngeal pouches and clefts. The endoderm of the pouches gives rise to, in order, the structures indicated in Table 7.

Pouch	Structure formed
1st pouch	Pharyngotympanic cavity Auditory tube Eustachian tube
2nd pouch	Tongue Palatine tonsils
3rd pouch	Thymus Inferior parathyroid gland
4th pouch	Superior parathyroid gland (C cells)

answers

Pouch	Structure formed
4th–5th pouch	Ultimobranchial bodies (parafollicular cells)

Table 7: Pharyngeal pouches

The thyroid gland originates from epithelial proliferation in the floor of the primitive pharynx and *not* from the larynx or branchial arches. It is connected by the thyroglossal duct to the foramen caecum at the junction of the anterior two-thirds and posterior third of the tongue. Ectopic thyroid tissue occasionally causes cysts along the path of the duct. The thyroid migrates to its final position in front of the tracheal rings. The parafollicular (C) cells come from the ultimobranchial body, a derivative of the 4th pharyngeal pouch.

Extended Matching Answers

43 Theme: Branchial arches

1 **A – First arch – anterior two-thirds of the tongue**
   C –Third arch – posterior third of the tongue

2 **A – First arch – anterior two-thirds of the tongue**

3 **G – Third pouch – thymus and inferior parathyroid gland**

Abnormalities of the branchial arches are caused by the following:

- Thyroid gland
  - Developed from the endodermal pouch
  - Arises from the 1st and 3rd arches
  - The thyroid gland migrates inferiorly and fails to descend completely

- Pierre Robin sequence
  - Due to a small retroverted tongue, cleft and palate abnormality, micrognathia, posterior larynx and obstructed breathing. This may be due to damage to the 1st branchial arch.

- Lateral cervical cyst
  - Used to be termed a branchial cyst
  - Results from an abnormality of the pharyngeal pouch, which involutes.

- Treacher Collins syndrome
  - Evolves due to damage to the 1st arch
  - Causes mandibular facial dysostosis
  - Associated learning difficulties.

- DiGeorge syndrome
  - Absent thyroid and parathyroid glands.

44 Theme: Impaired fetal lung development

1 **D – Potter's syndrome**

2 **F – Jeune's syndrome (asphyxiating thoracic dystrophy)**

3 **H – Dystrophia myotonia**

Impaired fetal lung development is seen in Potter's syndrome, Jeune's syndrome and dystrophia myotonica. It is not found in the infants of insulin-dependent diabetic mothers or in Duchenne muscular dystrophy. Impaired fetal lung development is not found in bronchiolitis, facioscapulohumeral dystrophy, Pickwickian syndrome or Kartagener's syndrome.

Embryology of the lung is also important with respect to stridor, which is associated with laryngomalacia and worsens from birth. If associated with a viral infection, the stridor worsens during the acute phase of the illness. Vascular rings around arteries and not veins cause acute stridor. They may be demonstrated by a barium swallow, on which an indentation of the oesophagus by the ring is noted. A diaphragmatic hernia is often noted and is most common on the left. Persistent pulmonary hypertension of the newborn is due to an abnormality of the pulmonary arteries that arise from the 6th branchial arch. The main pulmonary artery from the left 6th branchial arch and subdivisions arise from the left and the right arteries. The fetal pulmonary arteries are more muscular than those of the infant and therefore allow blood to be diverted from the lungs in fetal life. This may also lead to persistent pulmonary hypertension of the newborn.

Jeune's syndrome (asphyxiating thoracic dystrophy) presents with lung hypoplasia and poor cartilage development.

Dystrophia myotonia is often diagnosed in the infant by observing the mother's handshake and facial appearance. It is associated with polyhydramnios due to poor fetal swallowing, and thus poor lung development.

45 Theme: Development of the genitalia

1 **A – Coelomic epithelium, C – Sertoli cells, H – Mesonephric duct**

2 **B – Mesenchymal cells, G – Paramesonephric duct**

3 **D – Allantois, E – Urachus, F – Mesonephros,
J – Develop in the 10th thoracic level**

Organogenesis in the fetus begins around the 3rd week after conception (3/40) and is completed by the 8th week (8/40). This embryonic period

answers

denotes the highest risk of fetal abnormality. The development of the genital system begins at around 6 weeks after fertilisation (6/40). At this time:

- There is formation of the allantois (out-pouching of the yolk sac), which is involved in the formation of: (a) the bladder, (b) blood within its walls in the first 8 weeks of life, and (c) the umbilicus.
- As the bladder develops, the extra-embryonic portion of the primitive allantois degenerates, leaving a thick tube – the urachus – and its blood supply, which becomes the umbilical vessels.
- After the birth, the urachus becomes a fibrous cord – the median umbilical ligament.
- Gonads from *both* sexes develop from the mesonephros.
- Both sexes in the early stages have two pairs of genital ducts – a mesonephric duct and a paramesonephric duct.
- In males, the paramesonephric duct involutes and the mesonephric duct forms the efferent ductules, the vas deferens, the seminal vesicles and the ejaculatory duct.
- In females, the mesonephric ducts involute and the resulting paramesonephric duct forms the uterine tubes, uterus and vagina.
- The coelomic epithelium differentiates into somatic sex cord cells, which in turn differentiate into Sertoli cells in males and follicular cells in females.
- The mesonephros forms gonads of *both* ovary and testes.
- The mesonephros forms the ureteric bud in *both* sexes. This bud develops into the ureters, calyces and collecting tubules.
- Differentiation of the sex cord cells is determined by the encoding gene on the Y chromosome. This encoding gene is the sex-determining region and produces the testis-determining factor.
- Further maturation and development of the Sertoli cells influence the development of the male genitalia.
- There is further maturation and differentiation of the mesenchymal cells into: (a) follicles, and (b) the genital ridge to become the ovary.
- The external genitalia develop from a pair of labioscrotal folds, a pair of urogenital folds and the anterior tubercles.
- The testes and ovaries both develop in the region of the 10th thoracic level.

Emergency Medicine

Multiple True/False Answers

46 None is true

Figure 1 outlines the treatment algorithm that should be used.

Figure 1 Treatment algorithm for children by first medical responders

Consider when there is a compatible history of a severe allergic-type reaction with respiratory difficulty and/or hypotension, especially if skin changes are present

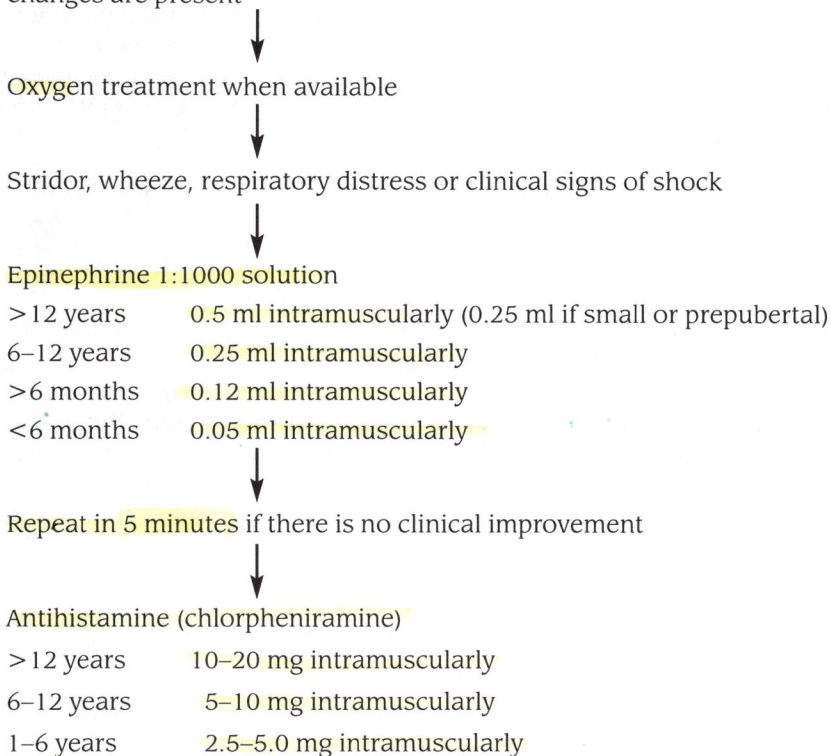

↓

Oxygen treatment when available

↓

Stridor, wheeze, respiratory distress or clinical signs of shock

↓

Epinephrine 1:1000 solution

>12 years	0.5 ml intramuscularly (0.25 ml if small or prepubertal)
6–12 years	0.25 ml intramuscularly
>6 months	0.12 ml intramuscularly
<6 months	0.05 ml intramuscularly

↓

Repeat in 5 minutes if there is no clinical improvement

↓

Antihistamine (chlorpheniramine)

>12 years	10–20 mg intramuscularly
6–12 years	5–10 mg intramuscularly
1–6 years	2.5–5.0 mg intramuscularly

answers

In addition, for all severe or recurrent reactions and patients with asthma, give hydrocortisone:

>12 years   100–500 mg intramuscularly

6–12 years   100 mg intramuscularly

1–6 years   50 mg intramuscularly

The alternative route for hydrocortisone is *slowly* via the intravenous route.

If the clinical manifestations of shock do not respond to drug treatment, give 20 ml/kg body weight of intravenous fluids. A rapid infusion or one repeat dose may be necessary.

An inhaled β_2-agonist such as salbutamol may be used as an *adjunctive* measure if bronchospasm is severe and does not respond rapidly to other treatment.

For profound shock judged IMMEDIATELY LIFE-THREATENING, give cardiopulmonary resuscitation/advanced life support if necessary. Consider a slow intravenous infusion of epinephrine 1:10 000 solution. This is HAZARDOUS and is recommended only for the experienced practitioner who can also obtain intravenous access without delay. Note the different strength of epinephrine that may be required for intravenous use.

Reference: Resuscitation Council (UK) *The Emergency Medical Treatment of Anaphylactic Reactions for First Medical Responders and Community Nurses*. Resuscitation Council (UK), London, 2002.

47 BCDE

The initial resuscitation dose of epinephrine (adrenaline) is 10 μg/kg. In cases of circulatory arrest thought to be due to circulatory collapse, a higher dose of 100 μg/kg can be given via the intravenous or intraosseous (i.o.) route. It is given every 3 minutes in all cases of cardiorespiratory arrest; that is, in all cases of asystole, pulseless electrical activity, ventricular fibrillation or pulseless ventricular tachycardia.

48 CDE

Calcium chloride and sodium bicarbonate are both irritants and could cause parenchymal lung damage. They are not lipid soluble.

The mnemonic LEAN is helpful in remembering the drugs that can be used via an endotracheal tube. LEAN represents lidocaine, epinephrine, atropine and naloxone.

Endocrinology

Multiple True/False Answers

49 ABCDE

The commonest form of CAH results from 21-hydroxylase deficiency, which has a reported incidence of 1 in 5000 in Europe, making it commoner than phenylketonuria.

An absence of the 21-hydroxylase enzyme means that there is overproduction of androgen hormones as the mineralocorticoid and glucocorticoid pathways are blocked (Figure 2). The same applies in 11β-hydroxylase deficiency. The effects of a deficiency of one of the enzymes arise from the loss of production of the distal hormone(s) and the stimulation of adrenocorticotrophic hormone because of this lack. This leads to an accumulation of the hormone occurring earlier in the pathway and the stimulation of production of related hormones.

In classic simple 21-hydroxylase deficiency, there is masculinisation of the female from an excess production of virilising hormones; in the salt-wasting form, there is also a deficiency of mineralocorticoid synthesis, with aldosterone deficiency as progesterone cannot be converted to deoxycortisone. This form presents with severe salt-wasting, excessive urinary sodium loss and dehydration, often during the neonatal period.

In 11β-hydroxylase deficiency, the picture is similar to that of classic 21-hydroxylase deficiency in terms of virilisation; this accounts for 5% of cases of CAH. However, owing to the accumulation of deoxycortisone, there is no salt-wasting; if the accumulation is excessive, there may be hypertension.

3β-Hydroxysteroid dehydrogenase deficiency leads to ambiguous genitalia; the excess of dehydroepiandrosterone and its conversion in tissues outside the adrenal glands leads to clitoromegaly in females. There is, however, insufficient virilisation potency to masculinise the male, hence the male neonate will have variable hypospadias and palpable testes. Owing to the defect in mineralocorticoid production, there is marked salt-wasting.

Figure 2 Androgen, mineralocorticoid and glucocorticoid pathways

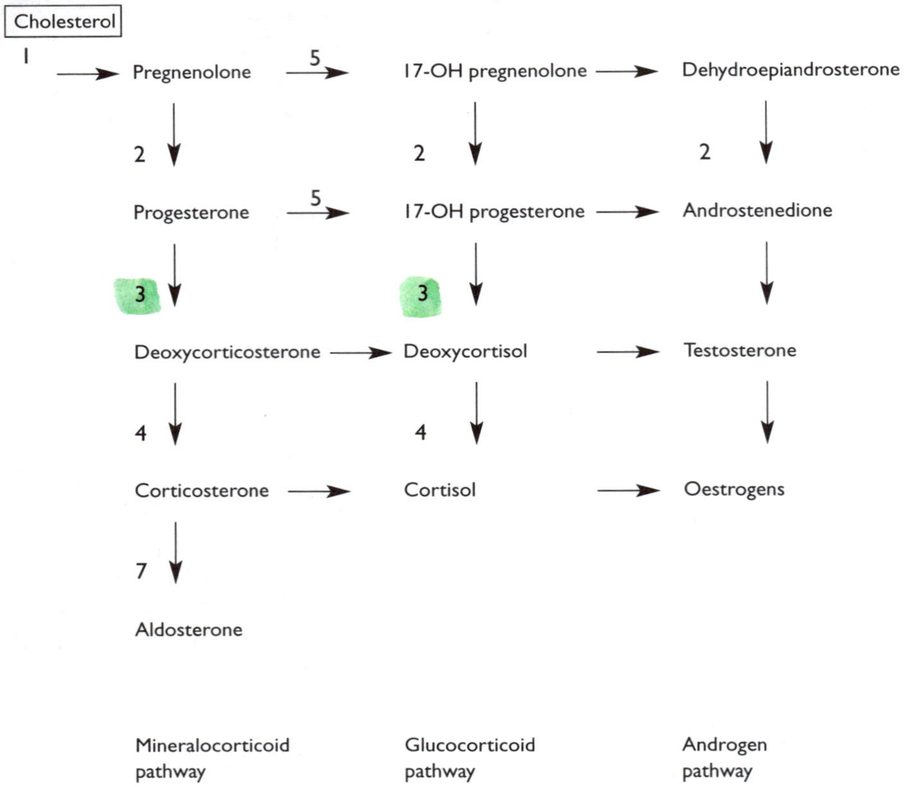

1 Cholesterol side-cleaving system
2 3 β-Hydroxysteroid dehydrogenase
3 21-Hydroxylase
4 11β-Hydroxylase
5 17α-Hydroxylase
6 17,20α-Lyase
7 18-Hydroxylase and 18-hydroxysteroid dehydrogenase
8 17β-Hydroxysteriod dehydrogenase

50 ABDE

Other forms of congenital adrenal hyperplasia that are associated with hypertension include17-hydroxylase deficiency and some cases of 11β-hydroxylase deficiency. Administered glucocorticoids are a commoner cause than Cushing's syndrome.

Best of Five Answers

51 C

The Tanner staging system is used to stage pubertal growth development. Three years prior to puberty, low levels of pulsatile luteinising hormone are found during sleep. The anterior pituitary secretes luteinising hormone and follicle-stimulating hormone in response to pulsatile gonadotrophin-releasing hormone from the hypothalamus. There is an increase in the amplitude and frequency of luteinising hormone as puberty approaches and the gonads increase in size. The average height gain in puberty is 30 cm (12 inches). In the UK, only 3% of males will have no signs of puberty at 13.4 years of age. During puberty, there is elongation of the eye and short-sightedness.

A disordered pattern of pubertal changes is termed dissonance and indicates an endocrinopathy. It is important to distinguish concordant from discordant pubertal development, ie gonadotrophin-dependent from gonadotrophin-independent disease. In males, the age of pubertal development is 11.5 years. Breast enlargement occurs in 40–60% of boys, which may cause social embarrassment, but in 10% it is due to a raised oestradiol level. Gynaecomastia is produced by the metabolism of testosterone and resolves within 3 years; it does not always need treatment. The ratings for stages of male puberty are as follows:

- Genital stage 1–5
- Pubic hair stage 1–5
- Axillary hair stage 1–3
- Testicular volume 2–25 ml (4 ml on average). Stage 4–5 is reached at approximately 13–14 years of age.

Peak height velocity occurs when testicular volume reaches 10–12 ml. A growth spurt occurs 2 years later in boys than in girls.

52 C

This child suffers from central precocious puberty, which occurs in females when puberty develops at under 8 years of age. True precocious puberty is ten times more common in females than males. Children usually present because of the development of secondary sexual characteristics. Gonadotrophin-dependent precocious puberty is a consequence of a premature activation of gonadotrophin pulsativity. This may be idiopathic and is constitutional in 80% of females. Almost all lesions are pathological in males. Causes of central precocious puberty may be human chorionic gonadotrophin-secreting tumours, including astrocytomas, ependymomas, gliomas, pinealomas, harmatomas, neurofibromas, hepatoblastomas, hepatomas and teratomas.

answers

53 C

In boys, delayed puberty is the absence of puberty by the age of 14 years of age. It is more common in males and is often constitutional, with a familial predilection. The delay in puberty may be due to a delay in the pubertal growth spurt and short stature, decreased height velocity, delayed adrenarche, delayed gonadarche and retarded bone age. Delayed puberty may be found in gymnasts, children suffering from chronic trauma, infection, irradiation or malignancy and in chronic rehabilitation after surgical procedures. Malignancies include craniopharyngioma, gonadal tumours and tumours of undescended testes. Hypothyroidism, Cushing's disease, anorexia, insulin-dependent diabetes mellitus and testicular feminisation may rarely present with delayed puberty. Syndromes associated with delayed puberty include 45XO, 45XXY, 47XXY, Prader–Willi, Laurence–Moon–Biedl and Kallmann's syndrome. Cyproterone acetate may rarely cause delayed puberty.

54 E

The causes of tall stature include familial, constitutional or endocrine disorders (precocious puberty, growth hormone excess, hyperthyroidism and congenital adrenal hyperplasia), homocystinuria and cirrhosis of the liver. Syndromes associated with tall stature include Marfan's syndrome, homocystinuria, Soto's syndrome, Klinefelter's, Fragile X and Asperger's syndrome, and Beal's contractural arachnodactyly. Beckwith–Wiedemann's syndrome produces large babies, not tall children. Hyperinsulinism causes macrosomia in the infant of a diabetic mother, but the effect weans off after 10 months of age so the children are of normal stature.

Extended Matching Answers

55 Theme: Obesity

1 **H – Prader–Willi syndrome**

2 **A – Laurence–Moon–Biedl syndrome**

3 **G – Constitutional obesity**

Childhood obesity appears to lead to adult obesity. It is found across all social classes and is associated with an above-average height in puberty. The protein leptin contributes to the regulation of body fat stores. Despite diet, exercise and behavioural management, fewer than 10% of patients may be treatable.

After smoking, obesity is one of the most preventable causes of death in the developing world. A body mass index (mass in kg/height in m²) of 29–32 is associated with an increased mortality of 60%. Even a small weight loss will decrease the mortality associated with insulin-dependent diabetes mellitus and hypertension. Associations related to an increase in body weight include early weaning, formula milk feeding, poor diet, behavioural abnormalities, depression, inactivity, immobility, tall stature, diseases associated with advanced bone age, early puberty, neurodevelopmental abnormalities and physical handicap.

Investigations may include measuring the height with a Harpenden stadiometer, bone age with a radiograph of the left hand (bone age may be advanced) and serum cholesterol level (which may be raised). Treatment options are limited but may include dexfenfluramine, an appropriate diet and surgery.

56 Theme: Short stature

1 **A – Familial short stature**

2 **B – Constitutional delay of growth and puberty**

3 **D – Spondylo-epiphyseal dysplasia**

Familial short stature is associated with short parents and a normal bone age, and is reversible. Constitutional delay of growth and puberty is associated with a decreased height and bone age, but after the pubertal growth spurt these children often catch up with their peers.

Skeletal dysplasias include spondylo-epiphyseal dysplasia, which is associated with a short trunk and a normal limb length. Other dysplasias include, camptomelic dysplasia (bent bones), achondroplasia and hypochondroplasia (short limbs, normal trunk).

Other causes of short stature include secondary growth failure (intrauterine growth retardation and low birthweight), delayed stature in puberty due to constitutional growth delay, chronic illness and hypothalamic, pituitary, gonadal and adrenal abnormality. Chronic illness, psychosocial deprivation and endocrine disorders are also associated. Syndromes associated include Laron, Mauriac's, Russell–Silver, Cockayne's, Noonan's, Turner's, Down's, Bloom's, Rubinstein–Taybi, Cornelia de Lange's, CHARGE, LEOPARD and DNA repair defects such as progeria. Fragile X syndrome does not cause short stature; in this the children are well known to be tall but become small adults.

ENT

Multiple True/False Answer

57 C

Serous (secretory) otitis media is symptomatic and may resolve spontaneously. It is often found in families in which the parents smoke. It may lead to learning difficulties, especially during the early years when hearing is essential for speech and language development. Breastfeeding appears to be protective.

Acute otitis media is prevalent during the winter months and is caused by bacteria, viruses and any obstruction to the eustachian tube. Bacteria include *Streptococcus pneumoniae* (50%), *Mycoplasma pneumoniae* and *Haemophilus influenzae*. *Staphylococcus epidermidis* and *Echinococcus granulosus* (dog tapeworm) are not associated. Antibiotic therapy appears to be effective in the majority of cases and may decrease the incidence of secondary complications, which include chronic suppurative otitis media, deafness, meningitis, mastoiditis and abscess formation. Other associations include lower socioeconomic class, cleft palate abnormalities, Down's syndrome, and Hunter's and Hurler's syndromes.

Best of Five Answer

58

1 **C – Nasopharyngeal intubation**

2 **E – Chronic obstructive apnoea**

3 **C – Pierre Robin sequence**

This child has Pierre Robin sequence, and the most appropriate immediate treatment is to maintain the airway to avoid obstructive apnoea and to insert a nasopharyngeal airway. Cleft lip and palate abnormalities are common, arising from non-development of the mesodermal tissue. The lips fuse between the 5th and 7th weeks of gestation, whereas the palate forms later between the 9th and 12th weeks. It is helpful to detect a cleft lip abnormality by 17 weeks' gestation. However, especially mucous clefts are more difficult to determine. The overall incidence of a cleft abnormality is between 1 in 700 and 1 in 2000 live births, with an individual incidence of 1 in 600 for cleft lip and 1 in 1000 for cleft palate.

The recurrence rate if a child has an affected sibling is 1 in 25. If one parent is affected, each offspring has a 1 in 20 chance of an abnormality. There is a 33% risk of an isolated cleft lip abnormality and a 25% increased risk of an isolated palate abnormality if there is a positive family history.

The aetiology of cleft lip and palate may be idiopathic, polygenic, environmental or due to medications (steroids or phenytoin) taken during the first trimester. Chromosomal abnormalities associated with cleft lip and palate include Patau's syndrome, Edwards' syndrome and Pierre Robin sequence. Mandibular hypoplasia associated with Pierre Robin sequence and Treacher Collins syndrome is found. Deafness is often also associated with Stickler's syndrome.

Extended Matching Answers

59

1 **D – Allergic rhinitis, E – Serous otitis media,
   H – Immunodeficiency**

Conductive hearing loss is recognisable by the prevalence of an air–bone gap. Bone conduction is noted by square brackets, and air conduction by an × or O symbol. There is normal bone and sensorineural transmission but an air loss at below –40 decibels. This is due to a problem between the outer and the middle ear. Conductive hearing loss shows a maximum of –60 to –70 decibels but no more. If the loss is greater than this, a sensorineural component to the hearing loss is found. A very wide air–bone gap of more than –45 decibels may be due to ossicular abnormalities. Causes include serous otitis media, hay fever, allergic rhinitis, craniofacial abnormalities, cleft palate and immune deficiency.

2 **A – Alport's syndrome, B – Gentamicin toxicity,
   C – Down's syndrome, F – Pendred's syndrome, I – Kernicterus**

Sensorineural hearing loss is found predominantly in boys, with an incidence of 1/1000. It is caused by a problem with the inner cochlea and/or central nervous system (auditory nerve, cochlear nerve, superior olive, lateral lemniscus or inferior colliculus). It is defined as unilateral or bilateral high-frequency hearing loss. High-frequency loss may be tested using oto-acoustic emission tests (eg brainstem evoked responses (BSER)). Bone conduction threshold tests bypass the outer and middle ear, and test the cochlear nerve and auditory nerve function. It excludes sensorineural deafness.

Causes are many; important ones include the following. Genetic, bilateral loss is found in Down's, Alport's, Pendred's, Cogan's and Romano–Ward syndromes. Perinatal complications include hypoxia, TORCH infections and kernicterus. Infections include mumps (unilateral) or flu-like or viral illnesses. Rare abnormalities include acute vertigo, labyrinthitis, vascular bleeding, trauma, head injury, intracranial tumours (posterior fossa tumour, acoustic neuroma and cerebellar tumour or pontinoma), cranial surgery, ototoxic drugs and craniofacial abnormalities.

3 **C – Down's syndrome, G – Turner's syndrome, J – CHARGE syndrome**

Mixed conductive and sensorineural hearing loss is very common and is often caused by a middle ear effusion. There is a wide air–bone gap as well as hearing loss at –80 dB. Syndromes often noted to suffer from the mixed type of hearing loss include Turner's, Down's and CHARGE syndromes.

Gastroenterology

Multiple True/False Answers

60 D

Bloody diarrhoea may be due to a viral, bacterial or protozoal infection (*Amoeba* for example). It is a notifiable condition (there being a public health requirement to do so), and the causative agent should be sought. Treatment is directed against the underlying pathogen, and treatment with loperamide is not recommended. Pathogens such as *Shigella* can elaborate an enterotoxin that can cause an encephalopathy. Amoebal infection can cause an amoebic abscess, which can rupture causing peritonitis.

61 None is true

Anal fissures are seen at all ages. A low dietary intake of fibre may be a predisposing factor in their development. This is a painful condition, often with fresh blood being seen on the stool or the lavatory paper. It is not clear that sphincterotomy is associated with the healing of anal fissures; it may be associated with incontinence in adults.

The natural course of anal fissures in children is that they heal spontaneously. The blood is bright red as it is fresh from the site of the anal fissure. Hard stool being passed stretches the anal ring and can cause splitting of this tissue, leading to blood loss. It may be associated in child sexual abuse cases; however, the vast majority of cases are due to constipation.

62 D

The mortality rate is as high as 1.55% of cases following perforation, but generally quoted figures are about 0.3% for simple cases. Wound infection is the commonest complication, being seen in between 5% and 33% of cases. Female fertility does not appear to be reduced in cases of perforated appendicitis. Spontaneous resolution has been reported in 8% of episodes.

63 B

Lactulose is associated with flatulence, abdominal pain and a significantly improved ease of evacuation and stool consistency from the baseline after 14 days of treatment.

Causes include hypothyroidism, associated syndromes such as Down's syndrome and Hirschsprung's disease, cystic fibrosis, anal fissures and dehydrating drugs. In the large majority of cases, however, no organic cause is found.

Cisapride has been shown to increase stool frequency in an outpatient setting, but it has been withdrawn owing to suspected adverse cardiac effects.

Chronic constipation can require extensive treatment, and the parents as well as the child need support and understanding. Half of all children in the preschool ages recover within 1 year and 66–70% within 5 years.

64 ABC

Helicobacter pylori is a Gram-negative, spiral, flagellated organism located in the stomach that is, in the majority of cases, acquired in childhood. It is believed to be causally related to the development of duodenal and gastric ulceration as well as gastric B-cell lymphoma and distal gastric cancer. It is estimated that 1 in 12 people with *H. pylori* infection will develop a peptic ulcer and 1 in 100 develop a gastric malignancy. In terms of alleviating the symptoms of gastro-oesophageal reflux, there does not seem to be a significant difference between eradicating *H. pylori* and placebo treatment.

65 None is true

Oral rehydration is as effective as intravenous fluid rehydration in terms of restoring blood electrolyte imbalances and is associated with a decreased duration of diarrhoea and time spent in hospital. The oral route is associated with weight gain when compared with intravenous rehydration. Worldwide, there are estimated to be between 3 and 5 billion cases in under-5-year-old children, the caused being viruses in 87% of cases in developed countries (with rotavirus the commonest agent).

66 ABCDE

Gastro-oesophageal reflux is caused by the transient or chronic relaxation of the lower oesophageal sphincter, giving rise to a passive transfer of gastric contents into the oesophagus. Vomiting, arching of the back in association with feeding, food refusal and failure to thrive are recognised complications. Less commonly seen are haematemesis, anaemia, cough, apnoea and wheeze. Risk factors include immaturity of the lower oesophageal sphincter, particularly in association with prematurity and in children with severe neurodevelopmental problems.

The majority of uncomplicated cases of reflux resolve by 12–18 months of age. Thirty per cent of cases associated with a hiatus hernia resolve by 4 years of age.

67 D

Infantile colic starts in the first few weeks of life and tends to cease by 6 months of age (the prevalence at 4–6 months being 7–11%). It is defined as excessive crying in a healthy child (hence is not caused by a urinary tract infection and is certainly not due to child abuse in 35% of cases!). A study has shown that 29% of infants aged between 4 and 12 weeks cried for more than 3 hours a day – general advice such as offering a dummy, using background soothing music and checking the nappy in comparison to carrying a child for longer than normal (normal being about 2 hours per day) showed no difference in duration of crying.

68 BCE

Jaundice, due to unconjugated hyperbilirubinaemia, that arises from breastfeeding (having excluded other organic causes) should not lead to the discontinuation of breastfeeding.

There is a risk of transfer of the human immunodeficiency virus from breast milk, although this is low in the developed world; the relative risks of using formula milk in the developing world (with unhygienic water sources and poor sterilisation) mean that breastfeeding should continue.

Lipid is composed of a large number of fatty acids, high in palmitic, oleic, linoleic and linolenic acids. Colostrum provides significant amounts of antibodies, which have a gut-protecting effect in the neonate.

Human milk is recommended for full-term infants during the first 6 months of life and ideally for the first year.

69 ABCDE

Causes can be divided into anatomical abnormalities, which are either congenital or acquired, and neuromuscular abnormalities.

Anatomical abnormalities:

- *nasal and nasopharyngeal*: choanal atresia, septal deflections, tumours
- *oral cavity and oropharynx*: cleft lip and palate, micrognathia, macroglossia and microglossia, inflammation of the mouth and pharynx, caustic lesions, pharyngeal diverticula
- *laryngeal*: stenosis, clefts, laryngomalacia
- *tracheal*: tracheo-oesophageal fistula, tracheotomy
- *oesophageal*: congenital abnormalities, infection, strictures and webs, achalasia, oesophageal dysphagia, cystic hygroma, craniofacial syndromes.

Neuromuscular abnormalities:

- *Central nervous system problems* (including cerebral damage from any cause): bulbar palsy, cranial nerve palsies, brainstem glioma
- *Peripheral nervous system:* traumatic, Guillain–Barré syndrome, laryngeal palsy
- *Autonomic nervous system:* familial dysautonomia (Riley–Day syndrome)
- *Primary disorders of muscle and the neuromuscular junction:* muscular dystrophy, myopathies, polymyositis, myasthenia, myotonic dystrophy, periodic paralysis.

70 ACD

This is a gluten enteropathy; the protein, gluten (the α-gliadin section), produces digestion-resistant substrates that are deamidated and presented via the human class II major histocompatibility complexes to be recognised by CD4+ cells. It is suggested that a 33-mer peptide is the key element to the origin of coeliac disease; this protein becoming exposed after digestion by gastric and pancreatic enzymes. Rice, oats and maize do not contain this homologous zone of 33-mer peptide and are not toxic in coeliac disease patients. The characteristic biopsy pattern is that of villous atrophy and crypt hyperplasia.

71 ABC

Other extraintestinal manifestations of inflammatory bowel disease include arthritis, and ocular and dermatological signs such as erythema nodosum.

72 C

With severe gastro-oesophageal reflux, failure to thrive is often an accompanying feature. All the other signs may be present.

73 ABCD

The blood pressure may be normal and the child is not yet in a moribund state (seen with a weight loss of over 15%). The mucous membranes will not be moist – the mouth will appear dry.

74 ABCD

Gilbert's syndrome is associated with an unconjugated bilirubinaemia, whereas all the other causes are associated with a conjugated hyperbilirubinaemia.

answers

75 A

Biliary salts are not required for the absorption of medium-chain triglycerides as they are rapidly broken down by lipase from the pancreas. The fatty acids of medium-chain triglycerides are 8–12 carbon atoms long and so are water soluble along with the products of lipase digestion. They are carried largely albumin bound and are metabolised in the liver.

Best of Five Answers

76 C

Marasmus is a form of protein calorie malnutrition which affects children less than one year of age and presents with diarrhoea, wasting and severe weight loss.

77 A

According to the WHO and the FAO definitions, protein calorie malnutrition may be classified accordingly:

	Weight (% of international standard)	Oedema weight/height	Deficient in
Kwashiorkor	60–80	+	+
Coeliac disease	<60	+	++
Marasmus	<60	–	++
Nutritional dwarfism	<60	–	Minimal
Underweight	60–80	–	+

Children with protein calorie malnutrition may be divided into two groups:

Marasmus

- <1 year of age
- Urban environment
- Early weaning onto dilute formula
- Recurrent gastroenteritis due to secondary lactose intolerance
- Wizened appearance, wasted with watery diarrhoea and decreased calorie intake
- Weight was <60% of the international standard
- Investigations show normal albumin, reduced thyroid function tests due to hyperproteinaemia.

answers

Kwashiorkor

- 1–4 years of age
- Rural environment
- Late weaning onto a low protein diet
- Learning defects later in childhood preciptated due to infections such as measles, malaria and gastroenteritis
- Appearance is flaky painted skin, apathy, flag sign (red hair), hepatomegaly, hyperthermia
- Weight <60–80% of international standard
- Normal calorie intake with reduced protein intake
- Investigations show hypokalaemia, hyponatraemia, hypoalbuminaemia, aminoacidurea, lactase deficiency and reduced thyroid function tests.

In both these categories there is marked reduction in subcutaneous fat, tissue and weight, as protein does not meet the demands of the body. There is normal head growth and a normal serum protein due to normal muscle breakdown. There is decreased calorie intake despite an increased carbohydrate and protein diet, and the total body water with respect to the body weight is increased. There is hypokalaemia due to decreased muscle mass and often hepatomegaly is associated with a fatty liver. Differential diagnosis includes intestinal tuberculosis, intestinal lymphangectasia, coeliac disease, food allergy and cystic fibrosis.

78 D

The classification given is classic for that of nutritional Ricketts due to phosphate deficiency brought about through unsupplemented cow's milk. Nutritionally there is inadequate intake of phosphate and vitamin D. This is the commonest cause of Ricketts in our population and in the 1920s was 30% of all A&E admissions. Recognised features of nutritional Ricketts include gross motor developmental delay, hypotonia and decreased muscle strength due to hypophosphataemia, craniotabes (soft skull, poor growth and bony deformity due to undermineralisation of the bone following vitamin D or 1,25-dihydrocholecalciferol deficiency). Other abnormalities notices are a decrease in phosphate with a normal or increased alkaline phosphatase and a normal calcium level. Disorders that cause Ricketts include:

Hepatobiliary disease
- Hepatocellular dysfunction
- Biliary atresia
- Cholestasis

Malabsorption
- Short gut syndrome
- Pancreatic insufficiency

Renal disease
- Hyperphosphataemic vitamin D resistant Ricketts
- Renal tubular acidosis
- Fanconi's anaemia
- Vitamin D dependent Ricketts type-I (1-alpha-hydroxylase deficiency) and glomerular diseases

Target cell abnormalities
- Vitamin D drug resistant type II disease

Tumours
- Non-ossifying fibroma
- Fibrous dysplasia or hemangiopericytoma

Medication
- Phenytoin

Extended Matching Answers

79 Calcium Metabolism

1 **A – Acute pancreatitis**

2 **A – Acute pancreatitis**

3 **D – Neither acute pancreatitis nor X-linked hypophosphataemic rickets**

4 **A – Acute pancreatitis**

Acute pancreatitis may present clinically with abdominal pain, vomiting, fever, Jaundice, ascites and a pleural effusion. The patient may present in shock. The correct cause is abdominal trauma; however, it may be due to:

A. Systemic illness, ie Henoch-Schönlein purpura, cystic fibrosis, Crohn's disease, systemic lupus erythematosus.

B. Viral infections, ie Coxsackie B, mumps, Epstein-Barr virus, hepatitis A, influenza A, as well as Mycoplasma.

C. Drugs, ie azathioprine, alcohol, diuretics, steroids.

In 50% of cases no aetiological cause is found. It may be induced by any cause of hypercalcaemia and hyperparathyroidism. Complications include hyperlipidaemia, high triglyceride and cholesterol levels, recurrent

answers

bacterial infections, biliary duct obstruction (pseudocyst formation), gallstones, duodenal obstruction and portal hypertension.

X-linked hypophosphataemic rickets (XLHP) is the most common cause of rickets in America. Males present as hemizygotes and are most severely affected than their counterpart heterozygote females. In XLHP the proximal convoluted tubule is damaged and fails to reabsorb phosphate adequately, resulting in hypophosphataemia and hyperphosphaturia. Aminoaciduria is no characteristic. The bloods results show a normal parathyroid hormone level and a normal calcium level. Treatment is with calcitriol (1,25-dihydroxy vitamin D) and phosophate supplements.

Genetics and Syndromes

Multiple True/False Answers

80 ADE

He has Prader–Willi syndrome. Other common phenotypic characteristics include brachydactyly, broad hands, epicanthic folds, a flat nasal bridge, hypotonia in the neonatal period, lax ligaments, a tendency to a decreased IQ, short stature and a widened first–second toe gap. Between 38% and 78% of children have hearing loss – this may be sensorineural, conductive or a mixture. About 50% have a congenital heart condition: atrioventricular septal defect in 45% of cases, ventricular septal defect 35%, isolated secundum atrial septal defect 8%, patent ductus arteriosus and tetralogy of Fallot in 4%.

81 BE

Alagille's syndrome comprises biliary hypoplasia, arteriohepatic dysplasia, hyperbilirubinaemia and vertebral and cardiac anomalies. Fifteen per cent of cases are autosomally dominant inherited with variable expression. Autosomal recessive inheritance and sporadic mutations are also found. It involves the deletion of p20 (*jag 1*) gene. A total of 20% of cases are premature/intrauterine growth retardation or small or small for gestational age infants. The aetiological factor may be a viral teratogenic factor.

Typical facial appearances include frontal bossing, a pointed chin, deep-set eyes and a prominent nose. Ophthalmological findings include posterior embryotoxin (70%) and pseudo-retinitis. Butterfly vertebrae (50%) are the known bony defects. Congenital heart disease is seen in 95% of cases, 10% of whom have cyanotic conditions and 50% of whom are known to have peripheral pulmonary artery stenosis. Liver complications include chronic cholestasis (paucity of the interlobar ducts), obstructive jaundice (often diagnosed when an infant), giant-cell hepatitis, pruritis and loose pale stools after the introduction of a fat-laden diet. Other

answers

clinical manifestations include learning difficulties, delayed sexual development and endocrine, neurological and renal abnormalities. The family cardiac history includes atrioventricular septal defect, hypoplastic left heart (HLH) and right ventricular outflow tract obstruction syndrome.

Diagnosis is aided by a HIDA liver isotope scan. Other useful tests include liver biopsy to exclude biliary atresia, ophthalmic assessment to review the cornea, cardiac assessment, a spinal radiograph to visualise the vertebral axis, a sweat test to exclude cystic fibrosis and finally a genetics assessment. The differential diagnoses include extrahepatic biliary atresia, hepatitis syndrome, hepatic thrombosis, cystic fibrosis, galactosaemia, tyrosinaemia and Zellweger's syndrome. The prognosis is satisfactory for 20–25% of cases, but the mortality rate due to liver failure is 3%.

82 None is true

All are minor criteria. Major criteria include:

- facial angiofibroma
- periungal/ungal fibroma
- shagreen patches
- hypomelanotic macules (more than three)
- cortical tuber
- subendymal nodule
- subendymal giant-cell astrocytoma
- multiple retinal hamartomas
- cardiac rhadomyosarcoma
- renal angiolipoma
- lymphangiomyomatosis.

Minor criteria are dental enamel pits, radial migration lines in the cerebral white matter and retinal achromic patches.

Two major features and one minor feature are required for a definite diagnosis of tuberous sclerosis.

Tuberous sclerosis is an autosomal dominant condition; the genetic loci involved are on chromosome 9q34 (*TSC1*) and chromosome 16p13 (*TSC2*).

83 E

All of the syndromes listed are associated with clinodactyly. Other associated syndromes include Russell–Silver's syndrome, trisomy 9p, trisomy 4p, trisomy 20p, XXXX syndromes and Down's syndrome. Clinodactyly may *occasionally* be seen in Wilms' tumour with associated aniridia, Prader–Willi syndrome and Williams' syndrome. It may be a normal characteristic.

84 B

Autosomal recessive inheritance is due to a single-gene mutation. The male:female ratio is 1:1. A child of heterozygote parents has a 1:4 chance of being affected.

Best of Five Answers

85 A

Genomic imprinting was first discovered in mice and subsequently found in humans. It is the inactivation of autosomal genes of either the paternal or the maternal genome. The problems are caused by DNA methylation. Here, the same genome is used differently depending on parental origin.

Two syndromes are often used to discuss genomic imprinting: Prader–Willi syndrome and Angelman's syndrome. Both conditions are caused by deletions of the same region of chromosome 15q12. A deletion of the paternally derived and inactivated genetic component of chromosome 15 results in Prader–Willi syndrome (whereby both copies are maternally derived). Likewise, a deletion of the maternally derived and inactivated genetic component of chromosome 15 results in Angelman's syndrome (in which both copies are paternally derived).

Uniparental disomy occurs when an individual has the correct number of chromosomes but has inherited both copies of one chromosome pair from one parent and no combination from the other. For example, if both copies of chromosome 15 are maternally derived (maternal uniparental disomy), there is an effective paternal deletion resulting in Prader–Willi syndrome. If, however, both copies of chromosome 15 are paternally derived (paternal uniparental disomy), there is effective maternal deletion resulting in Angelman's syndrome. Other disorders that show genomic imprinting include Beckwith–Wiedemann syndrome and Turner's syndrome.

86 C

Angelmann's syndrome is caused by a deletion on chromosome 15q11–q13. The disorder is due to the absence of the normal maternal copy of that 15q gene or paternal uniparental disomy for chromosome 15 (both copies of chromosome 15 being inherited from the father with NO COPY from the mother). Genomic imprinting is found in both Prader–Willi syndrome and Angelmann's syndrome. Trisomy rescue occurs when there is uniparental disomy and both copies come from both parents, causing a trisomy 15. This is not viable after conception. The above scenario would

answers

be indicative of Prader–Willi syndrome if there were an absence of the 15q gene as opposed to its presence. Other clinical manifestations of Angelmann's syndrome include brachycephaly and a puppet-like posture. The EEG is characteristic of this syndrome.

87 C

All of the options are chromosomal breakage disorders. Bloom's syndrome, however, is due to an autosomal recessive condition caused by a defect in the DNA repair mechanism. Bloom's syndrome is associated with the clinical phenotype described, and adult height rarely exceeds 145 cm. These children have severe sun sensitivity and are prone to recurrent infections. Due to a defect in the DNA repair mechanisms, these children are predisposed to malignancies. The phenotypic appearance of this child does not fit any of the other disorders listed.

88 D

Edward's syndrome results from trisomy 18 and has an incidence of 1 in 1000–3000. It is the second most common syndrome after Down's syndrome. It is termed an E group trisomy according to the Patau classification of groups A–G. Sixty per cent of cases die within 48 hours and 90% within the first year due to apnoeas. Cardiovascular abnormalities include atrial septal defect, ventricular septal defect and a persistent ductus arteriosus. There is no association with exophthalmos, but it may occur. Right choroid plexus cysts are found on coronal imaging, and 40–70% at post mortem are shown to have multiple large bilateral choroid plexus cysts (>10 mm). These may not become pathological but usually trigger an anomaly scan. Around 1% of cases may present with only a cyst, but 4% may present with other abnormalities.

Children with velocardiofacial syndrome have a classic facial appearance with hypertelorism, a tubular nose, a cleft lip/palate abnormality and cardiac anomalies. Children with Patau's syndrome usually present with midline defects and are less likely to have rocker-bottom feet. Children with Treacher Collins syndrome present with abnormalities of the branchial arches and pharyngeal pouches.

89 D

Fetal alcohol syndrome accounts for 10–20% of all children born with an IQ of <50–80. The incidence is 1 in 1000 live births, and the condition often presents with learning difficulties. The syndrome ought to be suspected in a mother who presents with memory loss and hypoglycaemia whose scans confirm intrauterine growth retardation with poor postnatal growth. Other late clinical features include poor concentration, inattention and fine motor incoordination. Cardiovascular abnormalities in 40% of cases include atrial septal defect and ventricular septal defect. Investigations should include chromosomal analysis, human immune deficiency virus status, syphilis, *Chlamydia* screening and an echocardiogram. The above are all differential diagnoses for fetal alcohol syndrome. 18q deletion syndrome should also be excluded.

Turner's syndrome is a common genetic disorder with chromosomal rather than mendelian inheritance. Mosaicism is the most common form, in 30%, with a chromatin-positive analysis. Barr body-negative and chromatin-negative patterns do exist. In all forms, the paternal sex chromosome is lost. If the Y chromosome is present, as in mosaicism, one must exclude 45X and 46XY as there is a high predisposition to gonadal neoplasia, so the ovaries must be removed to remove this highly associated risk. Children with Turner's syndrome have a phenotypic appearance similar to that of Noonan's syndrome. However, they also have generalised lymphoedema, with associated neck webbing. They have different cardiac abnormalities, including coarctation of the aorta, bicuspid aortic valve, aortic stenosis and total anomalous pulmonary venous drainage. They may have multiple renal abnormalities, sexual infantilism and growth failure with resultant short stature. They have multiple orthopaedic abnormalities and pigmented naevi. Like Noonan's syndrome, they may also suffer from ptosis, squint, bilateral otitis media and hearing loss.

Rubinstein–Taybi's syndrome has the phenotypic appearance of microcephaly, slanted palpable fissures, hyperplasia of the maxilla and mandible, and anteverted nares. The child may have learning difficulties and short stature. Flat broad thumbs and toes may be seen, and cataracts may be observed on fundoscopy.

Phenylketonuria can be diagnosed only once the child has been fully established on milk feeds. The phenotype is NOT suggestive of Marfan's syndrome.

90 D

Potter's syndrome is often associated with oligohydramnios, and the fetal ultrasound scan at 20 weeks often confirms small kidneys bilaterally. After delivery, there is often respiratory difficulty secondary to hypoplastic lungs. The child has characteristic facies with low-set ears, a beaked nose and micrognathia. A postnatal renal ultrasound scan confirms bilateral renal agenesis, and renal failure often occurs. Other conditions that are associated with fetal abnormalities include tracheo-oesophageal atresia (polyhydramnios) and maternal insulin-dependent diabetes (cardiomyopathy, septal hypertrophy, sacral agenesis). Siblings with anencephaly and in utero infections including toxoplasmosis, cytomegalovirus, rubella, syphilis, varicella zoster viral infections and congenital infections all require a detailed fetal anomaly scan. Fetal abnormalities are not associated with HIV, paternal insulin-dependent diabetes mellitus, influenza, hepatitis A or infectious mononucleosis.

91 E

The diagnostic criteria for neurofibromatosis are two or more of the following:

- Six or more café-au-lait spots
- Two or more neurofibromata (of any type) or one or more plexiform neurofibromas
- Axillary or groin freckling.

The incidence of neurofibromatosis is 1/2500. It is autosomal dominantly inherited, although 50% of cases arise from germ cell mutations. The *NF1* gene is a large gene, spanning over 350 kb of chromosome 17q11.2.

Café-au-lait spots are seen in 95% of cases; 70% have axillary or groin freckling. Neurofibromas include discrete dermal neurofibroma located within the dermis; nodular fibromas can arise at any peripheral nerve and can grow to a large size, for example the thoracic paraspinal dumbbell tumour. Plexiform neurofibromas grow on long portions of nerves, causing disfigurement and pressure effects on other tissues. Malignant change to peripheral nerve sheath tumours is seen.

Optic gliomas are seen in 15% of patients with the *NF1* gene, and 95% of these patients go on to develop benign melanotic hamartomas of the iris called Lisch nodules. Phaeochromocytomas are also seen in 0.1–5.7% of cases. Carcinoid syndrome has also been associated with *NF1*.

NF1 patients tend to have short stature and macrocephaly, with learning disability present in over half of the cases.

92

1 **A – Wilms' tumour with hemihypertrophy**

2 **C – Beckwith–Wiedemann's syndrome**

Beckwith–Wiedemann's syndrome results from an abnormality on chromosome 11p15. It is associated with islet cell hyperplasia. Children have an increased risk of developing other neoplasms, namely renal cortical adenoma, hepatoblastoma (right sided) and neuroblastoma (non-ballotable). There is a higher incidence of Wilms' tumour with hemihypertrophy. Medulloblastoma is less likely to be associated with Beckwith–Wiedemann's syndrome.

Extended Matching Answers

93 Karyotype abnormalities

1 **B – Chronic granulocytic leukaemia**

2 **E – Huntington's chorea**

3 **I – Patau's syndrome**

4 **H – Edwards' syndrome**

5 **D – Pierre Robin sequence, G – Meningomyelocele, J – Phenylketonuria**

6 **A – Burkitt's lymphoma**

The karyotype of an individual describes the number, size and shape of the chromosomes in the cell. The karyotype is best described in terms of aspects of various diseases:

1 Burkitt's lymphoma – this involves a translocation between chromosomes 8 and 14. A breakpoint in the chromosome 8 is inserted with the immunoglobulin heavy chain of chromosome 14. The Epstein–Barr virus is implicated in this process.
2 Chronic granulocytic leukaemia – 90–95% of cases are found to be positive for the Philadelphia chromosome formed by the reciprocal translocation of part of the long arm of chromosome 22 to chromosome 9.
3 Cri du chat syndrome.
4 Huntington's chorea – this autosomal dominant disease is a gene defect with an abnormality of the CA locus on chromosome 4. New mutations are, however, rare.
5 Klinefelter's syndrome.
6 Patau's syndrome (trisomy 13).
7 Edward's syndrome (trisomy 18).

A karyotype *cannot* be established for diseases such as meningomyelocele, phenylketonuria or Pierre Robin sequence.

94 Forms of inheritance

1 **A – Hereditary spherocytosis, B – Holt–Oram syndrome, E – Neurofibromatosis types I and II, I – Noonan's syndrome**

2 **C – Congenital adrenal hyperplasia, F – Friedreich's ataxia, G – Sickle cell anaemia, J – Xeroderma pigmentosum**

3 **D – α1-Antitrypsin deficiency, H – β-Thalassaemia**

Inheritance may be categorised into autosomal dominant, autosomal recessive and co-dominant inheritance.

answers

Autosomal dominant inheritance is a common form of inheritance that shows complete penetrance, although non-penetrance does occur. Roughly 1500 diseases are known in this category. The sex incidence is not equal, but the sexes are equally likely to be affected. Affected individuals are heterozygotes for the relevant defective gene. The risk of transmission is 1 in 2; ie 50% are affected and 50% show a normal phenotype. An unaffected person cannot transmit the gene disorder. If a parent has a normal genetic make-up, there is still a 50% chance of transmission to future pregnancies, and the risk for each pregnancy is the same. If both mother and father are affected, 50% of the offspring will be at risk of receiving the defective gene. The disease may also skip a generation.

Other associations with autosomal dominant inheritance include: achondroplasia, adult polycystic kidney disease, Allagille's syndrome, Alport syndrome, Crouzon's syndrome, DiGeorge syndrome, Ehlers–Danlos syndrome, familial hypercholesterolaemia, familial polyposis coli, facioscapulohumeral dystrophy, Gardner's syndrome, Gilbert syndrome, hereditary angio-oedema, hereditary elliptocytosis, hereditary haemorrhagic telangiectasia, hereditary obstructive cardiomyopathy, Huntington's chorea, hyperlipidaemia type II, malignant hyperthermia, Marfan's syndrome, myotonia congenita, myotonic dystrophy, osteogenesis imperfecta, Peutz–Jeghers syndrome, porphyrias (except congenital erythropoietic porphyria), pseudohyperparathyroidism, retinoblastoma, tuberous sclerosis, unilateral deafness, von Hippel–Lindau syndrome and von Willebrand's syndrome.

Autosomal recessive inheritance is the result of a single-gene mutation. Spontaneous mutation is exceptionally rare. There is often no previous history of the disease. The male:female ratio is 1:1. A child of two heterozygote parents has a 25% chance of being a homozygous subject. Here, the heterozygote is unaffected and a carrier state therefore exists. The frequency of carriers is greater than that of those with the disease, the carrier rate being 1 in 25. If both parents are affected, there is a 2 in 3 chance of being an affected carrier but only a 1 in 4 chance of being affected. Homozygote subjects will have affected children only if the partner is also a homozygote or a heterozygote for the condition. If an affected individual marries a genetically normal person, all the children will become carriers. The incidence rate is therefore 1 in 2500. Autosomal recessive conditions are more common within consanguineous marriages.

Other diseases with autosomal recessive inheritance include agammaglobulinaemias, albinism, ataxia telangiectasia, β-thalassaemia, Bloom's syndrome, Cockayne's syndrome, congenital erythropoietic porphyria, Crigler–Najjar type I syndrome, cystic fibrosis, cystinuria, Stevens–Johnson's syndrome, familial Mediterranean fever, Fanconi's anaemia, Gaucher's disease, glucose-6-phosphate dehydrogenase deficiency, haemochromatosis, homocystinuria, inborn errors of metabolism, infantile polycystic kidney disease, Laurence–Moon–Biedl syndrome, limb girdle muscular dystrophy, mucopolysaccharidoses (except Hunter's syndrome), Niemann–Pick disease, oculocutaneous albinism, Pendred's syndrome, sickle cell anaemia, Tay–Sachs disease, thanatophoric dwarfism and Wilson's disease.

Associations of co-dominant inheritance include β-thalassaemia and α1-antitrypsin deficiency.

95 Anticipation

1 **B – Fragile X syndrome (type A), C – Friedreich's ataxia, E – Myotonic dystrophy**

2 **D – Spinocerebellar atrophy type I, F – Huntington's chorea, G – Spinomuscular atrophy**

3 **A – Marfan's disease, H – Cystic fibrosis, I – Homocystinuria, J – Kartagener's syndrome**

Genetic anticipation occurs when successive generations are more severely affected by a disease process and at a younger age. The increase in severity of the disease is caused by an increase in the number of trinucleotide repeats, a trinucleotide repeat being a sequence of relevant genetic material that is expanded to contain up to thousands of repeating DNA base pair triplets. The repeats disrupt the protein configuration and cause disease. This methylation of the gene, which is the process of increasing the trinucleotide repeats, is abnormal and interferes with the excision of the introns.

The severity of disease expression is related to the size of the gene, and the gene increases in size when it is passed from parent to child. This phenomenon is best displayed by a slight increase in the trinucleotide repeats (permutation) in the maternal or paternal great-grandmother. It is often quiescent in the maternal grandmother. The disease manifests itself in the *next* generation male. In neurodegenerative conditions, there are rarely more than 150 trinucleotide repeats, with little anticipation. A patient with more than 1000 repeats will have severe disease, whereas if there are fewer than 400 the disease is less severe. Diseases that show anticipation can be divided into two categories (Table 8).

Category 1:	a	Diseases that are repeated in an *untranslated region*
Untranslated	b	There is *much* somatic variation
	c	The nature of the repeat *varies*
	d	The phenotype *varies*
	e	The expansion is often *extreme*, ie 50–1000 repeats
	f	Anticipation is *severe*

answers

g   Diseases are *maternally* inherited:
    myotonic dystrophy
    Fragile X syndrome (type A)
    Friedreich's ataxia

Category 2: Translated	a	Diseases repeated in the *translated* region
	b	There is *little* somatic variation
	c	All have the *CAG* trinucleotide repeats
	d	They all encode *glutamine*
	e	The expansion is *moderate*, ie 40–100 repeats
	f	Anticipation is *modest*
	g	Diseases include:
		Huntington's chorea
		Spinomuscular atrophy
		Spinocerebellar atrophy

Category 3: Negative	Cystic fibrosis, Marfan's disease, homocystinuria and Kartagener's syndrome do not show trinucleotide repeat anticipation

Table 8: Categories of anticipation

96 Theme: Pedigree maps

1   **B – Autosomal recessive inheritance**

2   **D – X-linked recessive inheritance**

3   **A – Autosomal dominant inheritance**

Pedigrees can be simple to work out if a few rules are understood. It may be useful to take a systematic approach such as:

1   Count how many males and females are affected and obtain a ratio.
2   If the ratio is 1:1, the condition is autosomal dominant or autosomal recessive.
3   If the ratio shows females>males, there is X-linked dominance, ie father-to-daughter transmission.
4   If no females are affected, it is X-linked recessive.
5   If there is male-to-male transmission, the condition is autosomal dominant or rarely autosomal recessive, but never X-linked dominant.
6   If there is a history of intrauterine death, stillbirth or neonatal death, consider an autosomal recessive condition.
7   If the condition has arisen out of the blue, it is autosomal recessive.

Five extra points may help in differentiating the different types of inheritance:

• Autosomal recessive and autosomal dominant inheritance can transmit from male to female, ie both son and daughter can be affected?

answers

- Consanguineous marriages may result in autosomal recessive diseases.
- X-linked recessive diseases – mothers transmit to sons and with a 50% chance to daughters.
- X-linked dominant diseases – mothers transmit to sons or daughters with a 50% chance.
- X-linked dominant diseases – fathers cannot transmit to sons and affect daughters.

Remember that when no pattern fits this, maternal mitochondrially inherited diseases should be considered.

97 Theme: X-linked inheritance

1 **C – Vitamin D-resistant rickets, E – Goltz syndrome, F – Incontinentia pigmenti, G – Orofacial digital syndrome**

2 **A – Ichthyosis, B – Retinitis pigmentosa, D – Severe combined immune deficiency, H – Alport's syndrome, I – Fragile X syndrome, J – Lesch–Nyhan syndrome**

3 **None**

X-linked dominance is a rare form of inheritance that affects both sexes but women more than men. All the children (ie 100%) of affected homozygous females are affected. The carrier females pass the trait to 50% of their sons and 50% of their daughters. All the daughters of the affected males are affected but none of the sons. The sons may be affected in utero, but they display a lethal form of the disease and may not survive, ie they are miscarried or stillborn. Therefore only females appear to be affected. Other diseases that show X-linked dominant inheritance include the XG blood group.

X-linked recessive inheritance is described for more than 200 conditions. This form of inheritance is more common in males. The affected males usually carry the gene, and homozygous males are very rare. There is no male-to-male transmission; the affected cases have affected brothers and maternal uncles. Fifty per cent of sons are affected, and 50% of daughters are carriers. The risk of transmission from carrier female to male child is 1 in 2, and there is the same risk that the daughters of carrier females will be carriers themselves. The gene is passed on by carrier female to affected son. An affected male can only have a normal son and a carrier daughter. The mother is not always a carrier. There is no maternal age effect. X-linked recessive inheritance is a chromosomal disorder and not a single-gene defect. Females may therefore show some features through lyonisation, and have variably severe manifestations as a result of random inactivation.

Other X-linked recessive disorders include Alport's syndrome, Becker's muscular dystrophy, Fabry's disease, chronic granulomatous disease,

answers

colour blindness, complete testicular feminisation, congenital sideroblastic anaemia, Duchenne muscular dystrophy, haemophilia A and B, Hunter's syndrome, ichthyoses, glucose-6-phosphate dehydrogenase deficiency (fauvism), Lowe's syndrome, nephrogenic diabetes insipidus, ornithine transcarbamylase deficiency, pseudohypoparathyroidism, Wiskott–Aldrich syndrome, X-linked adrenoleukodystrophy, X-linked agammaglobulinaemia, X-linked ocular albinism and X-linked recessive hyperphosphataemic rickets.

98 Theme: Genetic pedigree

1   **J – 10%**

2   **B – 2%**

3   **A – 1%**

The pedigree displays Robertsonian genetics: 45XX (t)21:14. The Robertsonian translocation occurs between acrocentric chromosomes 13, 14, 15, 21 and 22. The long arms fuse at their centromeres. The total fused complement is that of 45 chromosomes, but the translocation is balanced as the child still has a full genetic make-up. A balanced translocation (carrier) may in theory give birth to a chromosomally imbalanced offspring. If a child is found to have an unbalanced translocation, there is a 25% risk that that parent has a balanced Robertsonian translocation and a 75% risk that it is de novo. The balanced chromosome produces a normal phenotype, whereas the unbalanced chromosome produces dysmorphism. The following are found: normal phenotype 1:4, monosomic abortion 1:4, balanced translocation 1:4, Down's syndrome 1:4 with a 2 in 3 chance of Down's syndrome. There is a 10% carrier rate for the mother, a 2–2.5% carrier rate for the father and a 1% chance of mosaicism. The risk of a sibling being affected is only significant if the mother has a balanced translocation. A carrier has >10% chance of recurrence occurring if she is a (t) 21:14 carrier. Carrier fathers rarely have affected children.

99 Theme: Genetic syndromes

1   **H – Williams' syndrome**

Williams' syndrome is also termed idiopathic infantile hypercalcaemia. The abnormality is found on the 7q chromosome. It may present as a familial or sporadic trait. The abnormality involves a mutation of the elastin gene and the adjacent genes. These children have mild learning difficulties and are able to cope, with verbal and social skills. They have delayed motor and peripheral skills, and an average IQ of 50. Cardiovascular abnormalities may also include aortic stenosis, peripheral pulmonary stenosis and supravalvular aortic stenosis. The differential diagnosis must include vitamin D toxicity, distal renal tubular acidosis, idiopathic hypercalcaemia, hypercalciuria, immobilisation, hypothyroidism, hypoxaluria and cortical nephrocalcinosis.

2   D – Fragile X syndrome

Fragile X syndrome is neither autosomal dominant nor autosomal recessive. It is a condition with non-classical mutations that are unstable and produce a genetic disease. Some of these mutations lead to unusual non-mendelian inheritance. De novo mutations are rare, and this disorder is mainly X-linked with an abnormality on the fragile site of the distal end of the long arm of chromosome at XQ27.3. Approximately 45% of the DNA will have fragile cells on the karyotype when grown on folate-deficient medium. When the gene breaks, the child lacks expression of the gene so the condition is familial. This disorder shows allelic expansion of a trinucleotide repeat sequence (CGG) in the *FMRI* gene (familial retardation gene) on the X chromosome. The trinucleotide repeat increases with each generation. The initial mutation may start with an unaffected male. The female transmission increases with each repeat until the change becomes significant and the fragile X occurs. This disorder displays lyonisation. Carrier females are clinically unaffected, but 10–33% of female heterozygotes will have learning difficulties (the exception to the rule).

3   F – Smith–Lemli–Opitz syndrome

Smith–Lemli–Opitz syndrome is a metabolic disorder. An abnormality in the breakdown of cholesterol due to cholesterol reductase deficiency causes a low cholesterol level. Investigations show a decreased cholesterol level with an increase in 7OH-CO-cholesterol. There are two types of clinical presentation: types 1 (major) and 2 (minor). Treatment includes a diet high in cream and eggs, which will improve the personality problems but will not alter the learning difficulty.

100 Theme: Genetic syndromes

1   A – Noonan's syndrome

Children presenting with Noonan's syndrome may show normal chromosomes, with a normal karyotype but of variable expression. It may present as a single autosomal dominant gene abnormality or it may be a sporadic familial disorder. Direct transmission from an affected parent to the child occurs in 30–70% of cases. The incidence is 1 in 1000–2500 live births. It is more common in boys than girls, and they may look phenotypically similar to children with Turner's syndrome but do not have the karyotype. The abnormality is an intragenic deletion. The gene has been mapped to chromosome 12q. He cannot have Turner's syndrome as he is male.

2   **C – Patau's syndrome**

Trisomy 13 is caused by an unbalanced translocation and has an incidence of 1 in 5000–10 000. The prognosis is extremely poor, with infants rarely surviving beyond 4–6 months of age. Midline craniofacial defects include holoprosencephaly, midline cutis aplasia over the vertex of the skull, and a cleft lip and palate abnormality. Cardiac defects occur in 80% and may include ventricular septal defect, atrial septal defect or a persistent ductus arteriosus. Renal abnormalities occur in 60% and may present with abnormal external genitalia. Limb abnormalities are as stated above, and eye abnormalities include cataracts, colobomata, microphthalmia and corneal opacities.

3   **B – Laurence–Moon–Biedl syndrome**

Laurence–Moon–Biedl syndrome is an autosomal recessive disorder that presents with the above clinical phenotype. Other features include polydactyly, night blindness, knock-knees, obesity and tinnitus.

Haematology

Multiple True/False Answers

101 ABCDE

Drugs that inhibit the enzyme cyclo-oxygenase, such as aspirin and non-steroidal anti-inflammatory agents, inhibitors of phosphodiesterase, for example dipyridamole. Antibiotics such as penicillin and cephalosporin, heparin and alcohol alter platelet function. Primary marrow disorders such as acute leukaemias and myeloproliferative disorders are also a cause; bypass surgery similarly disrupts platelet function.

102 ABCE

Microangiopathic causes include HUS, thrombotic thrombocytopenic purpura, meningococcaemia and disseminated intravascular coagulation. Mechanical causes are seen in patients with cardiac valves or arterial grafts, or who enjoy long-distance walking (march haemoglobulinuria). Infections such as malaria and clostridia, and chemical and physical causes including burns, may also cause fragmentation of the red cells. Liver disease and renal disease are also associated with disrupted red blood cells.

103 DE

There is an inability to make haemoglobin A, hence the levels of HbF and HbA$_2$ are increased and there is an expansion of medullary tissue, so frontal bossing is common. This is associated with bone thinning and therefore an increased frequency of fractures. Hepatosplenomegaly is invariably present due to extramedullary haemopoiesis, and anaemia is a key component. Treatment includes regular transfusion and the avoidance of iron overload by using desferrioxamine.

Best of Five Answers

104 E – Glucose-6-phosphate dehydrogenase deficiency

105 D – X-linked recessive

This X-linked recessive condition is not exclusive to males and involves both homozygous females and heterozygous males. Heterozygous females have two populations of cells and therefore show a variable degree of clinical expression of the disease. There are 50 variants but two types of glucose-6-phosphate dehydrogenase deficiency, known as:

- the African type – a mild variant found in 10–20% in those presenting from Africa
- the Mediterranean type – a severe variant in which 10–25% present from those who live in the Mediterranean, Middle East, Papua New Guinea and South-east Asia.

The disease is also found in north and central America in the Negro population. It is an important cause of jaundice amidst the Chinese population. There are four clinical syndromes described in glucose-6-phosphate dehydrogenase deficiency:

1 drug-sensitive haemolytic anaemia
2 favism
3 neonatal jaundice
4 congenital non-spherocytic haemolytic anaemia.

Type II favism is an acute intravascular haemolysis and occurs 6–24 hours after the ingestion of fava beans or the inhalation of pollen. Drug-sensitive haemolytic anaemia is caused by the effect of the drug on intrinsically abnormal red blood cells that are unable to maintain normal glutathione levels so that the oxidative medication can cause an acute haemolytic episode. Drugs responsible include sulphonamides, nitrofurantoin, chloramphenicol, quinine, primaquine, chloroquine, dapsone, methylene blue, naphthalene, vitamin K, aspirin, phenacetin, co-trimoxazole, probenecid and PAS. Penicillin and tetracyclines do not cause favism.

106 B – Evans' syndrome

Acute idiopathic thrombocytopenia (ITP) is a common disorder with an incidence of 4/100 000. It usually presents in children between the ages of 2 and 4 years, with an equal ratio of boys to girls. There is an increased incidence during the winter and spring, often preceded by an upper respiratory tract infection. It is thought to be due to the immune-mediated destruction of platelets by the coating of platelets with antiplatelet antibody. The majority of cases resolve spontaneously.

The child presents with a prodromal coryzal illness, purpura, mucosal bleeding and pallor. There is no associated lymphadenopathy, and often a spleen seen on scanning is rarely palpable. An enlarged spleen usually suggests another diagnosis. If autoimmune haemolytic anaemia and ITP coexist, Evans' syndrome is described, which includes purpura, bruising, recurrent nosebleeds, gastrointestinal bleeds and melaena. Splenomegaly and fundal haemorrhages are unusual unless there is severe anaemia.

107

1 **C – Parvovirus B19**

2 **D – Hereditary spherocytosis**

3 **D – Spheroidal cells**

4 **A – Autosomal dominant**

This child is suffering from hereditary spherocytosis. There is an increased permeability of the red blood cells and an increase in red blood cell energy expenditure from glycolysis to maintain the shape of the red blood cell. There is therefore an abnormality of the cytoskeleton of the red blood cell membrane and in the protein spectrum, which is a component of the cell wall. The membrane is abnormally permeable to sodium ions, leading to an influx of up to 50% of sodium ions. Spherocytes are more rigid than healthy red blood cells and are destroyed in the spleen, causing an associated splenomegaly.

There is a congenital and an acquired form of this disorder. The diagnosis is confirmed mainly by the presence of spherocytes on the blood film, a bone marrow biopsy is often requested, with ring sideroblasts noted after splenectomy, and there is aplastic anaemia. The osmotic fragility test shows increased haemolysis, although this is not specific to hereditary spherocytosis and is therefore infrequently used. (The folate level may be reduced with an increase in the iron and ferritin levels.) Children with hereditary spherocytosis show a low level of haptoglobins, which confirms intravascular haemolysis as the child's haemoglobin binds to the haptoglobins and is excreted. Because of the increase in iron level and the normal electrophoretic pattern, there is no iron deficiency anaemia or thalassaemia.

The differential diagnosis includes disorders that may show spherocytes on the blood film, namely autoimmune haemolytic anaemia, *Clostridium welchii* infection, severe burns and a blood transfusion reaction. A further diagnosis to consider in a neonate is ABO incompatibility.

answers

Extended Matching Answers

108 Theme: Resuscitation fluids

1   **C – Disseminated intravascular coagulation**
    D – Thrombotic thrombocytopenic purpura
    G – Persistent bleeding (high prothrombin time)
    I – Surgery to the biliary tract

2   **A – Hypoalbuminaemic oedema**
    B – Nephritic syndrome
    F – Major burns
    H – Liver disease

3   **J – Factor 2, 5, 7 and 9 deficiency**

Fresh frozen plasma (FFP) is derived from blood or plasma. It has a long shelf-life and may be stored at −30°C. It contains clotting factors, anticoagulants, immunoglobulins, chloride esterase inhibitor, α1-antitrypsin, albumin, blood group antibodies and fibronectin. Double-volume FFP has recently been found to be helpful in reducing recipient donor exposure and is available in 300-ml aliquots. The blood group must be observed when giving FFP. Blood group AB is the 'universal donor' for FFP. If factor 2, 7, 9 and 10 are not available, FFP may be given. FFP is also indicated in the treatment of an increased prothrombin time, which may be noted in patients on warfarin therapy. FFP may be used for reversal in warfarin overdose; there is instant correction to overwarfarinisation associated with bleeding. FFP is not the first-line therapy for factor deficiencies as the relevant factor should be given if the patient is deficient. If, however, no factor is available, FFP may be given.

109 Theme: Clotting profiles

1   **D – Von Willebrand's disease**

2   **E – Co-dominant**

Von Willebrand's disease is the most common congenital bleeding disorder in childhood. It shows co-dominant inheritance, the abnormality being found on chromosome 12. The disorder is worse in the homozygous form, ie in the children of consanguineous parents. The incidence is 3–4/100 000 children. The disorder results from the underproduction of von Willebrand's protein, which is responsible for platelet aggregation and the carriage of factor 8. Von Willebrand's protein has three functions: it protects factor VIII in the circulation; it aids platelet adhesion to the endothelium; and it prolongs the bleeding time and in so doing decreases the FC component of the VW antigen and its function. There are three types of von Willebrand's disease:

- type I – classical (autosomal dominant)
- type II – moderate (autosomal dominant)
- type III – severe (autosomal recessive).

In the severe type, there is a total qualitative lack of protein. No protein is present, and no factor VIII or von Willebrand's factor is found. This has a poor prognosis.

110 Theme: Pancytopenia

1   **A – Aplastic anaemia**
    B – Paroxysmal nocturnal haemoglobinuria
    D – Acute myeloid leukaemia
    F – Haemosiderosis
    G – Drug-induced marrow aplasia
    I – Miliary tuberculosis

2   **C – Acute lymphoblastic leukaemia**
    E – Gaucher's disease
    H – Stage IV neuroblastoma
    J – Severe haemolytic-uraemic syndrome

3   **C – Acute lymphoblastic leukaemia**
    E – Gaucher's disease
    F – Haemosiderosis
    H – Stage IV neuroblastoma
    J – Severe haemolytic-uraemic syndrome

There are many causes of pancytopenia, including paroxysmal nocturnal haemoglobinuria, acute myeloid leukaemia, miliary tuberculosis, folic acid deficiency, vitamin B12 deficiency, systemic lupus erythematosus, hypersplenism and drug-induced marrow aplasia, all of which may be reversible. Causes of pancytopenia with associated splenomegaly include low-grade non-Hodgkin's lymphoma, acute lymphoblastic leukaemia, rhabdomyosarcoma, stage IV neuroblastoma, severe haemolytic–uraemic syndrome, severe thrombocytopenia purpura, and vitamin B12 deficiency. Pancytopenia with hepatosplenomegaly is seen in cirrhosis of the liver and Gaucher's disease. Haemosiderosis and aplastic anaemia do not characteristically cause pancytopenia with splenomegaly.

111 Theme: Methaemoglobinaemia

1   **C – Primaquine**
    D – Nitrates
    E – Potassium chlorate
    F – Quinones
    H – Chloroquine

answers

2   **G – Ascorbic acid**
    J – Methylene blue

3   **A – Paraquat**
    B – Vitamin D

Methaemoglobinaemia may be congenital or acquired. This child has acquired methaemoglobinaemia after taking malarial prophylaxis and ingesting nitrates used in the water supply on her farm in Gloucestershire. This may occur when oxidative drugs are ingested and cause oxidation of the haemoglobin. Other drugs that may cause methaemoglobinaemia include paracyanide, sulfasalazine, nitroglycerine, nitrites, sulphonamides, analine dyes, lignocaine, prilocaine and chromates. The following are not associated with haemoglobinaemia: Paraquat and home central heating with a blocked flue (which causes carbon monoxide poisoning). Treatment for acquired methaemoglobinaemia includes vitamin C, methylene blue and ascorbic acid.

HIV/AIDS

Multiple True/False Answers

112 ABCE

HIV is transmitted by needle-stick injury, sharing drug-giving paraphernalia, the infusion of infected blood products and unprotected heterosexual and homosexual intercourse. Vertical transmission also occurs. HIV refers to infection with either type 1 or type 2 virus. There is characteristically a variable period of being asymptomatic followed by repeated episodes of illnesses of varying severity.

113 BCD

Triple therapy is associated with a reduction of 50% in the risk of death in HIV-infected patients and is believed to be less likely to give rise to resistance. People with sexually transmitted diseases are at greater risk of HIV infection, but presumptive mass treatment has not been found to decrease the incidence of infection.

114 AE

Longer courses of zidovudine are more effective at reducing transmission, nevirapine being more efficacious than zidovudine. The presence of p24 antigen or culture-positive samples indicating viraemia is associated with a doubling of the risk of vertical transmission. Breastfeeding is also a risk and is not recommended in developed countries. The risk in developing countries is not as great as the risk of making up formula feeds. Three-quarters of infants die without treatment in the first year of life.

The risk of vertical transmission varies in different countries:

- Europe: 15–20%
- USA: 15–30%
- Africa: 25–35%.

HIV type 2 is rarely transmitted vertically; HIV type 1 infection occurs during pregnancy, in the intrapartum period or by breastfeeding.

answers

115 AB

Treatment with aciclovir is associated with a reduction in mortality at different stages of HIV infection.

116 CE

Co-trimoxazole has no effect on dealing with infection by viral infections or fungal infections or *Pneumocystis carinii* pneumonia.

Immunology

Multiple True/False Answers

117 AC

The pathogens associated with an underlying immune disorder are:

- mycobacteria – type 1 cytokine defects
- Gram-negative bacteria – neutrophil defects
- enterovirus – antibody defects as well as defects in cell-mediated immunity
- *Staphylococcus* – neutrophil defect
- *Meningococcus* – complement deficiency
- *Pneumococcus* and *Haemophilus influenzae* B – antibody and complement defects
- *Salmonella* – type 1 cytokine defects and cell-mediated defects
- *Mycoplasma* – antibody defects
- herpes viruses – defects in cell-mediated immunity.

118 ABDE

The exact underlying defect in chronic cutaneous candidiasis is still poorly understood; there is, however, poor T-cell proliferation and cytokine production. There is persistent *Candida* infection, which is recurrent and not eliminated by antifungal treatment. Oesophageal involvement can lead to gastro-oesophageal reflux and dropping off the weight centiles. In over 50% of cases, there is, in the second to third decade of life, an endocrinopathy that may involve combinations of hypoparathyroidism, Addison's disease, pernicious anaemia, hypothyroidism and diabetes mellitus.

119 ABCDE

Intravenous immunoglobulin treatment will negate the live virus. The other categories bestow vulnerability and could lead to evolution of the disease. Post-transplant children are maintained on lifelong immunosuppression.

120 C

A decreased C3 level is seen in:

- Systemic lupus erythematosus (antinuclear antibodies (ANA), anti-double-stranded DNA)
- Mesangiocapillary glomerulonephritis
- Membranoproliferative glomerulonephritis (type 2)
- Post-streptococcal glomerulonephritis
- Infective endocarditis
- Infected ventricular shunts
- Chronic Gram-negative infection.

Increased complement activation is seen in:
- Hereditary angioneurotic oedema (C1 inhibitor deficiency)
- Pregnancy
- Paroxysmal nocturnal haemoglobinuria
- Glomerulonephritis grade 2.

The level is not changed in focal sclerosis, focal segmental glomerulonephritis, Henoch–Schönlein purpura or haemolytic-uraemic syndrome.

A defect in the complement system **should** be suspected in:

- Focal swelling after trauma
- Recurrent meningococcal infection (C5–C9) (encapsulated organisms)
- Recurrent staphylococcal infection
- Lupus-like syndrome (major histocompatibility complex, chromosome 6).

Complement abnormality is **not** suspected in recurrent folliculitis, *Pneumocystis carinii* infection (combined immunodeficiency) or delayed separation of the cord (leukocyte adhesion defect), or inherent complement deficiency in membranoproliferative disorders. Pancreatitis involves the consumption of normal levels of complement.

Best of Five Answers

121 D

Leukotrienes are synthesised by leukocytes and mast cells. They mediate inflammation and allergic reactions in the following ways:

- By increasing neutrophil/eosinophil chemotaxis and vascular permeability, and inducing smooth muscle constriction
- By causing arteriolar constriction and bronchoconstriction.

Leukotriene D4 is identified as the slow-reacting substance of anaphylaxis (SRS-A) and is responsible for smooth muscle contraction. Leukotrienes are derived from arachidonic acid and not palmitic acid. The arachidonic acid is cleaved into cyclooxygenase derivatives, which produce prostaglandins, prostacyclins and thromboxanes. The other pathway produces leukotrienes. Leukotrienes do not act synergistically with SRS-A as leukotrienes are produced by mast cells to dampen the inflammatory response and decrease granulocyte formation at the site of invasion.

122

1   **E**
2   **B**
3   **BCDE**

X-linked agammaglobulinaemia is the most common immunoglobulin deficiency. The gene is localised to the long arm of the X chromosome, with the abnormality being in the gene for the B-cell tyrosine kinase. It is more common in males. This disorder is associated with an increased risk of blood malignancies. It presents after 3–6 months of age when the level of IgG resulting from in utero placental transfer has decreased. The child presents with recurrent bacterial infections in the first 2 years of life, namely lung and sinus infections. Causes of hypogammaglobulinaemia include:

1   Common variable immune deficiency
2   Hypogammaglobulinaemia with raised IgM (X linked)
3   Transient immune deficiency of infancy.

Prenatal diagnosis is possible. Investigations show a profound failure of B-cell development so plasma cells from the bone marrow are absent. There is an abnormal B-cell function and number so there are isohaemagglutinins or surface immunoglobulins. Investigations undertaken include those stated, including finding an increase in OKT3 (49–63% of cases). Neutrophil, lymphocyte, PHA, nitroblue tetrazolium (NBT), sweat test and T-cell function are all normal. The PHA test measures T-cell proliferation. The T-cell lymphocytes are identified by their ability to form rosettes with sheep red blood cells. T-cell proliferation gives the total percentage of lymphocytes; the number is increased if no B-cells are present. Monoclonal antibodies are now used to identify and characterise T-cells. Monoclonal antibodies against T3 receptors measure the total T-cell number, T4 receptors, the T helper cell population and T8 receptors in the T suppressor/cytotoxic (Ts/c) group. Treatment includes prophylactic antibiotics and intravenous immunoglobulins. Bone marrow transplantation is carried out if medical interventions fail.

answers

123

1 **E**

2 **B**

This autosomal recessive disorder occurs due to dysfunctional and reduced natural killer cells. Pathologically, the leukocytes contain giant cytoplasmic granules. Other cells can also contain these granules, giving features of the disease. Melanocytes do not, however, disperse pigments within the cells; hence there are features of partial albinism. There are no hyperpigmented lesions of the lumbosacral area. Schwann cells are affected, causing sensory and motor neuropathies. People with this disorder have an increased susceptibility to infections due to defective chemotaxis, degranulation and bactericidal activity of the neutrophils. There is an increased incidence of malignancies and a high mortality rate with respect to infection.

Affected children present with ataxia, seizures, muscle weakness and an illness similar in picture to lymphoma with lymphotrophic viruses, eg Epstein–Barr virus. Ocular symptoms include nystagmus, photophobia and an increased red reflex.

Investigations depict a decreased antibody-dependent cell-mediated cytolysis of the tumour-like reaction. There is decreased function of natural killer cells, a prolonged bleeding time, impaired platelet aggregation, decreased neutrophil number and a pancytopenia when associated with bacterial and viral illnesses.

124

1 **C**

2 **E**

3 **B**

4 **B C**

Chronic granulomatous disease may manifest soon after birth with superficial skin sepsis and painful regional lymphadenopathy. Lesions heal incompletely with sinus formation. Due to the inability to kill catalase-positive micro-organisms, chronic deep infections occur, and common recurrent skin abscesses with *Staphylococcus*, *Escherichia coli*, *Serratia*, *Klebsiella* and *Candida* may be seen. Less common infections include those involving *Shigella*, *Salmonella* and *Pseudomonas*. All these pathogens display a lack of oxidative respiratory burst and produce oxygen free radicals. The neutrophil is unable to activate one or more oxidases to consume oxygen to produce superoxide or hydrogen peroxide following phagocytosis. Superoxide stimulates the hexose monophosphate shunt, and halides are produced. The interaction of reactive oxygen molecules, myeloperoxidase and halides with phagocytic vacuoles results in the effective killing of catalase-containing bacteria. Gram-negative rods and catalase-negative organisms are killed normally as they generate hydrogen peroxide. *Aspergillus* is a common secondary pathogen, but herpesvirus is not found as a pathogen. Other clinical manifestations include respiratory tract infections, sinusitis, urinary tract infections, obstructive uropathy and liver infections (abscesses) with hepatosplenomegaly. Gastrointestinal involvement includes necrotic granulomas, colitis, oesophageal strictures, perinatal abscess and pyloric strictures. Chronic osteomyelitis of the small bones of the hands and feet may be difficult to treat. The differential diagnosis includes neutrophil-killing defects, Chédiak–Higashi syndrome, lactoferrin deficiency, mobility disorders such as lazy leukocyte syndrome and Shwachman syndrome. Chronic illnesses, including systemic lupus erythematosus, rheumatoid arthritis, tuberculosis, toxoplasmosis, hyper-IgE syndrome and malnutrition, may also be associated.

125 E

Hereditary angioneurotic oedema is caused by a deficiency or a defect in C1 esterase inhibitor protein, the amount found being <25% the normal value. The protein modulates the intravascular activation of complement, and its deficiency leads to angioedema. There is an inability to synthesise normally functioning C1 inhibitor. The condition is genetically inherited in an autosomal dominant fashion. This disorder usually presents in late childhood or adolescence, ie aged 10–20, when attacks become more frequent. Hereditary angioneurotic oedema causes 2% of all angioedemas. It is found that 85% of individuals have very low levels of inhibitor and 15% have normal or raised non-functioning protein; this may therefore be used in a functional assay. This disorder involves the deeper layers of the skin.

Clinically, hereditary angioneurotic oedema presents with:

- Abdominal pain and cramps due to swelling of the intestinal tissues secondary to visceral oedema
- Subcutaneous oedema and swelling (72 hours maximum)
- Laryngeal oedema (presenting as a hoarse voice and sometimes causing fatal obstruction); these may be unresponsive to antihistamines
- Symptoms related to phases of the menstrual cycle
- Triggers including a prodromal rash, skin trauma (as the protein involved is within the fibrin cascade), menstruation and emotional stress.

There is no urticarial rash or inflammation suggestive of pruritus.

Investigations

During an attack, C4 and C2 levels are decreased. There is an excessive stimulation of C2, C4 and related vasopeptides, due to uninhibited

answers

activity of complement. The deficiency of C1 inhibitor permits C1 to continuously cleave its substrates C4 and C2 to cause them to become deficient. The C1 and C3 levels are normal, as is the number of B cells. C2b splits off to become the vasoactive component.

Treatment

Treatment used to date includes anabolic steroids, to increase protein levels. This prevents acute attacks, and the symptoms resolve in 2–3 days. Fresh frozen plasma and C1 esterase concentrate are used in the acute phase to restore normal levels of inhibitor. Androgen agonists, ie danazol or stanozolol, are used in the chronic phase. The side-effects of danazol include androgenic problems in childhood. Other drugs used include alpha-aminocaproic acid and tranexamic acid. Steroids, adrenaline and antihistamines are not effective.

126. D

T-cell deficiency	B-cell deficiency	Neutrophil defect
Wiscott–Aldrich syndrome Ataxia telangiectasia	Bruton's disease	Chronic granulomatous disease

Primary immunodeficiencies are:

- X-linked agammaglobulinaemia
- Hyper-IgG syndrome
- Severe combined immunodeficiency syndrome
- Wiskott–Aldrich syndrome
- Ataxia telangiectasia
- DiGeorge syndrome
- Hereditary angioneurotic oedema.

Antibody/B cells	Bacteria
T cells	Viruses, especially herpes simplex, cytomegalovirus (CMV), Epstein–Barr and herpes zoster Mycobacteria, especially live in macrophages *Candida*
Complement (rare)	Impaired C5–C9 complex of the complement cascade Bacteria (meningococcal) Lytic terminal complement pathway
Phagocytes	Bacteria, especially in those immuno-compromised or undergoing cancer chemotherapy Fungi

Table 9: Infections found and type of associated immune deficiency

Extended Matching Answers

127 Theme: Complement receptor abnormalities

1 A
2 I
3 B
4 J
5 H
6 C
7 A
8 E
9 F
10 D

The following table summarises the complement proteins and the diseases with which they are associated.

Pathway	Complement protein	Disease(s)
Classical	C1q, C1R, C2, C4	SLE, glomerulonephritis
Alternative	D	Recurrent neisserial infections
	Properdin	Non-recurrent meningococcal infections
Lectin	Mannose-binding lectin (MBL)	Susceptibility to infections (otitis media)
C3 deficiency syndrome	C3, factor I, factor H	SLE, severe infections, glomerulonephritis
Membrane attack	C5, C6, C7, C8, C9	Recurrent neisserial infections
Complex control proteins	C1 inhibitor, delay accelerating factor (DAF), homologous restriction factor (HRF)	Hereditary angioneurotic oedema
Complement receptor	CR3	Recurrent pyogenic infections

Table 10: Complement proteins and the diseases with which they are associated

C1 activity is increased in C1 inhibitor deficiency. C3a, C4a and C5a all have the ability to bind to mast cells and leukocytes to trigger the release of histamine and mediators. They are involved in anaphylaxis, vasodilatation, swelling and inflammation, bee-sting anaphylaxis and extrinsic allergic alveolitis. C5a is a potent neutrophil chemotactic agent that promotes macrophages to CR1 and CR3 receptors to neutralise. C3a mediates the suppression of antibody responses. C3b enhances cell-mediated toxicity and solubilisation of the immune complexes. Low C3 and CH50 levels correlate strongly with a very poor outcome in patients with multiorgan failure. C5b enhances the antibody response involved in the chemotaxis of neutrophils, monocytes and eosinophils. Individuals with a deficiency of C5 are at an increased risk of developing meningococcal sepsis.

The membrane attack complex (C5–C9)

The membrane attack complex (MAC) assembles following the cleavage of C5 to form C5b via the classical or alternative pathway. It inserts into cell membranes to form a channel that traverses the membrane and leads to cell lysis. Its binding to cells is inhibited by very low-density lipoprotein, and autologous cells contain membrane control proteins that partially protect them from the action of MAC. MAC is active only against autologous cells. Paroxysmal nocturnal haemoglobinuria is caused by a decreased number of control membrane proteins so there is an increased sensitivity to MAC.

Complement receptors

These receptors participate in various functions of the host defence system, including the C1 and C4 neutralisation of viruses. There are four complement receptors:

CR1: found in leukocytes in tissues and the circulation. It has a role in immune complex handling and is decreased in SLE as an acquired defect.

CR2: important in the lymphocyte reaction with other cells. Epstein–Barr virus may act as a ligand.

CR3 and CR4: form a receptor that also includes IFA-1 (a lymphocyte receptor). If the level of this receptor is decreased, pyogenic infection results as the neutrophils are unable to bind the bacteria coated in C3. Cryoglobulinaemia displays a low C4 but a normal C3 level.

128 Theme: Human leukocyte antigens

1   **F**
2   **E**
3   **C**

HLA DR/W2, DR/W3 and B8	Systemic lupus erythematosus
HLA B8/DR3	Dermatomyositis herpetiformis
HLA DR5/DR2	Kaposi's sarcoma
HLA DR3	Chronic active hepatitis, Graves' disease, myasthenia gravis, Addison's disease and Sjögren's syndrome, idiopathic membranous nephropathy, systemic lupus erythematosus
HLA DR2	Goodpasture's syndrome, narcolepsy, multiple sclerosis, juvenile insulin-dependent diabetes mellitus
HLA DQW2, DR3/7	Coeliac disease
HLA A3/B14	Idiopathic haemochromatosis
HLA A28	Schizophrenia
HLA B5	Behçet's disease and arthritis of inflammatory bowel disease (IBD) (ulcerative colitis)*
HLA B27	Ankylosing spondylitis, psoriatic arthropathy**, Reiter's disease, reactive arthritis***
HLA DR4	Rheumatoid arthritis
HLA DR5	Hashimoto's disease, pernicious anaemia
HLA B35	Subacute thyroiditis
HLA DR2, 3, 4	Insulin-dependent diabetes mellitus
HLA A1, B8, DR3	Linkage equilibrium in nephrotic syndrome, acquired immunodeficiency syndrome (AIDS)
*IBD arthritis	10% of IBD sufferers get arthritis. Some get ankylosing spondylitis associated with HLA B27
**Psoriasis	May show a weak HLA B27 link
***Reactive arthritis	After *Salmonella*, *Shigella*, *Yersinia enterocolitica*, *Camplyobacter* and Reiter's disease, ie causes of bloody diarrhoea

Table 11: HLA associations

answers

129 Theme: Hypersensitivity

1 **D (graft-vs-host disease)**
2 **C (Henoch–Schönlein purpura (HSP))**
3 **E (Graves' disease)**

There are six types of hypersensitivity:

Type 1 – This is an immediate and often anaphylactic reaction involving IgE, IgG4, mast cells and basophils. It involves a vasodilatory response, activation of eosinophils and leukotrienes, and the release of vasodilators such as histamine, serotonin and bradykinins. Histamine is a spasmogen, causing bronchial smooth muscle contraction. A wheal and flare is formed. The process is involved in:

- Atopic disease
- Asthma
- Hay fever (pollen)
- Eczema
- Anaphylaxis
- Food and drug intolerance
- Bee and wasp stings.

For the purpose of exams, remember that sodium cromoglicate stabilises the mast cell membrane.

Type 2 – This is cell-bound hypersensitivity, which is antibody dependent and involves the cytotoxic cells. Here, circulating antibody (IgG and IgM) binds to cell–cell surface antigen receptors and activates complement, which causes cell lysis/damage and macrophage opsonisation with neutrophil activation. This type of hypersensitivity is involved in:

- Graves' disease
- Haemolytic anaemia
- Myasthenia gravis
- Idiopathic thrombocytopenic purpura (ITP)
- Goodpasture's syndrome
- Hyperacute graft rejection
- Reduction of ABO incompatibility
- Role in cancer
- Blockage of antibody.

Type 3 – This involves circulating immune complexes and is complement mediated. It is activated via IgG and IgA. There are three mechanisms for producing disease:

- The combined effects of low fever and a weak antibody response
- As a complication of autoimmune disease in which the continued production of antibody to self antigen forms complexes
- The formation of immune complexes at the body surfaces, eg in the lungs.

Type 4 – This involves the cell-mediated immune system. It involves a delayed T-cell-mediated reaction. It is associated with:

- Acute early rejection
- Graft-versus-host disease (late rejection)
- Rheumatoid arthritis
- Contact dermatitis
- Acute allergic alveolitis
- The reaction in tuberculosis with the tuberculin skin test (72 hours) and granulomatosis (21–28 days)
- The Heaf test response.

This delayed hypersensitivity is seen with:

- Sarcoidosis
- Malignant lymphomas such as Hodgkin's disease
- DiGeorge syndrome (absent or decreased T-cells)
- Corticosteroid treatment
- Leprosy (borderline)
- Malnutrition
- Wiskott–Aldrich syndrome
- Crohn's disease
- Extrinsic allergic alveolitis
- Schistosomiasis
- Extreme old age – it decreases with age
- It is **not** associated with the Arthus reaction.

Type 5 – This is stimulatory with IgG antibody, which results in:

- Long-acting thyroid stimulation, which causes the prolonged stimulation of thyroid hormone
- Graves' diseases and hyperthyroidism.

Type 6 – This class involves killer cells, which lyse targets coated with antibody, eg tumours or helminths.

Note: Types 7–10 do not exist.

130 Theme: Immunoglobulins

1   **B**
2   **D**
3   **A**

Immunoglobulins are composed of two heavy and two light chains. The heavy chain, with one variable and three to four constant regions, determines immunity. The light chains (kappa and lambda) each have one variable and one constant region. Papain (protease enzyme) cleaves immunoglobulin at the hinge region into two separate fragments, the Fab (antibody-binding) and Fc (crystallisation) fragments.

answers

The Fc portion (effector end) of an immunoglobulin molecule:

- Determines the half-life of the antibody and therefore the class of immunoglobulin
- Allows bonding to mast cells and macrophages
- Allows the bonding and activation of complement
- Does not provide antibody specificity (the antibody-binding end – variable region)
- Has the ability to transfer across the placenta
- Can activate the complement cascade (ie fixation).

IgG has two Fc portions; the Fc portions are determined by valency for antigen (IgM = 5, IgG = 2).

The Fab fragment (variable end) of the molecule is contained within the variable regions, VL and VH. In these domains lie the six hypervariable regions that determine antibody specificity.

All classes of immunoglobulin are monomers, excluding IgM which is a pentamer. IgA and IgM are polymers, IgA being a dimmer that has a secretory component. Only IgG and IgA exist as subtypes. There are two components to the formation of immunoglobulins. The classical component involves IgG1–2 and IgM; the alternative component compromises IgG4, IgA, IgD and IgE. J chains are associated with both IgA and IgM.

	IgG	IgM	IgA	IgD	IgE
Biological property	Secondary response	Primary response	Secretory	B-cell surface maker	Allergy anaphylaxis
Placental transfer	+	–	–	–	–
Complement fixation	+	+	–	–	–
Interaction with Fc on:	Classical	Classical	Alternate	–	–
Neutrophils	+	–	–	–	–
Eosinophils	+	–	–	–	+
B-cells	–	–	–	+	–
Lymphocytes	+	+	+	+	+
Mast cells	–	–	–	–	+
Plasma cells	+	–	–	–	–
Macrophages	+	–	–	–	+
Basic form	Monomer	Pentamer	Mon/dimer	Monomer	Monomer
Heavy chain	IgG 1–4	M	IgA 1–2	D	E
Subclasses	4	–	2	–	–
Molecular weight (kDa)	150 000	950 000	160 000–380 000	175 000	190 000
Sediment constant (S)	6.6	–	7/11	7	8
Carbohydrate content (%)	2–3	12	7–11	9–14	2
Valency for antigen	2	5 (10)	2/4	2	2
	IgG	IgM	IgA	IgD	IgE
Distribution in the intravascular space (m/s)	50	80	50	75	50
Half-life (days)	23	5.8	5.1	2.8	2.5
% of the immune pool	75	10	15	Trace	Trace

Table 12: Immunoglobulin properties

Infectious Diseases and Tropical Medicine

Multiple True/False Answers

131 CDE

The mortality rate varies in different countries: in the USA it is 1.4–7.0/100 000 and in Australia 0.5–1.2/100 000 for children aged between 1 and 11 years. The mortality rate is higher in adults, at about 31/100 000, varicella pneumonia being the commonest cause for admission. One randomised controlled trial showed that children with a malignancy had significantly less clinical deterioration than controls.

Early administration of aciclovir to healthy individuals can alleviate the symptoms.

132 ABCDE

Toxoplasma gondii is a parasite that may be transmitted by eating fruit or vegetables contaminated by infected cat faeces or by the ingestion of tissue cysts from raw meat.

During pregnancy, it may be transmitted transplacentally to the fetus; the earlier this occurs, the more complications are usually seen. These vary from intrauterine death to chorioretinitis, hydrocephalus, neonatal intrauterine growth retardation and other ocular defects. Disease may present at birth or at a later time with neurological or ophthalmological pathology.

133 C

The following periods are recommended:

- Chickenpox – 5 days from skin eruption
- *Escherichia coli* enteritis – 2 days of negative stool samples
- Fifth disease – no exclusion recommended as this is such a common illness
- *Haemophilus influenzae* infection – 48 hours after treatment has commenced

- Hepatitis A – 5 days in under 5-year-olds
- Infectious mononucleosis – no exclusion
- Influenza A – no exclusion
- Lyme disease – no exclusion
- Measles – 5 days from onset of the rash
- Meningococcal disease – 48 hours from the start of treatment
- Mumps – 5 days from the onset of parotitis
- Norwalk virus – 3 days from the last episode of diarrhoea
- Pertussis – 5 days from the start of treatment
- Roseola infantum – no exclusion
- Rubella – 5 days from onset of the rash
- Scabies – until treated
- Scarlet fever – 5 days from the start of treatment
- Streptococcal pharyngitis – no exclusion
- Tuberculosis – smear positive: 2 weeks after starting treatment; smear negative: no exclusion.

134 ABCDE

Influenza type A causes a worse illness than type B. The incubation period is 1–4 days, infected patients being contagious from the day prior to the onset of symptoms until 5 days after the onset. Elderly patients, children and those who are immunosuppressed are at greatest risk of being admitted (as well as of having one of the complications listed above).

135 ABCDE

Entamoeba histolytica is the enteral pathogen whereas *Entamoeba dispar* is a commensal. This was determined by sequencing of the ribosomal DNA of these organisms. The incidence of liver disease due to amoebiasis is disproportionately raised in young men, the reasons for which are not yet clear.

Invasion of the colon occurs, and diarrhoea, dysentery or bleeding by itself may be the clinical manifestation of bowel disease. Spread to the liver by way of the portal circulation occurs following invasion of the bowel wall. This liver abscess may present some time after the history of travel.

Liver abscess can rupture and cause pleuropulmonary amoebiasis through the diaphragm. This is thought to occur in 7–20% of patients; brownish sputum can be seen, particularly if a hepatobronchial fistula has formed. Less commonly, liver abscess can rupture into the peritoneum; this is associated with a sudden onset of shock and peritonitis. Even rarer is rupture into the pericardium. Mortality in this case is as high as 30%, the patient having either pericarditis or cardiac tamponade.

Amoebic serology has a high sensitivity (94%) and high specificity (over 95%) for the diagnosis of liver abscess.

answers

136 BCE

Lyme disease is caused by a spirochaete, *Borrelia burgdorferi*, in North America. It can also be due to *B. garinii* and *B. afzelii*. The vector for transmission is *Ixodes*, the tick that can be found with deer and rodents.

Some infected people remain asymptomatic, and spontaneous resolution frequently occurs. The condition is not commonly fatal but can be a cause of carditis, myocarditis, conduction defects, arthritis, erythema migrans, neuropathies, meningitis and encephalopathy. One randomised controlled study has shown that ceftriaxone improves arthritis compared with penicillin.

137 AC

The eradication of nasopharyngeal carriage is reduced by antibiotic treatment, but there is no evidence that this reduces the likelihood of disease. Risk factors include exposure to smoke and crowding, the greatest risk being in the first week following exposure to a contact case. The highest incidence is seen in preschool children, with a secondary peak incidence seen in adolescents.

138 AB

Xylitol is associated with abdominal pain so is not used in children.

The difference between 5- and 10-day courses are that the longer course significantly reduces treatment failure, relapse and reinfection rates at 8–10 days but shows no difference at 20–30 days.

Immediate treatment with antibiotics as compared with no treatment significantly reduces the number of days of earache and ear discharge, as well as the amount of paracetamol used after 1 day; there is, however, no difference in pain scores.

139 E

Measles, an RNA paramxyovirus, is spread by airborne droplets and is highly contagious. Neonates are protected by passive immunity from the in utero transfer of maternal antibodies. There is an incubation period of 10–12 days and a 2- to 4-day prodrome with upper respiratory tract symptoms and a high fever, with a widespread rash that lasts up to 5–6 days. Measles is associated with conjunctivitis, coryzal features and a dry, non-productive cough.

140 CD

There is no difference between the options for statements A, B and C.

Over one-third of the world's population is infected with *Mycobacterium tuberculosis*, which kills more people than any other infecting organism. Poverty, overcrowding, homelessness and inadequate health services, human immunodeficiency virus and immunosuppression are all risk factors.

141 CE

Children have tonsillitis more commonly than adults; the UK incidence in primary care is 1/1000 population every year. Bacterial swabs are only successfully cultured in a minority of cases; viruses may have a role to play in this condition, but there is a great deal of uncertainty surrounding their contribution. Peritonsillar abscess is a well-recognised sequel.

Best of Five Answers

142 C

Brucellosis is a zoonotic disease that is commonly acquired in the Mediterranean and the Middle East and has a 1- to 5-week incubation period. It is usually contracted by consuming unpasteurised milk and cheese products or when working on farms, in abattoirs or in butcher's shops with goats, sheep, pigs and cattle. The acute febrile stage shows a high fever, headache, malaise, profuse sweating and general arthralgia with a few localising signs. The chronic phase, which occurs in 20–60% of cases, presents with relapsing fever, sweats, arthralgia, malaise, anorexia, weight loss, constipation and emotional disturbance. Examination often reveals marked lymphadenopathy with a papular rash. Abdominal examination may reveal hepatosplenomegaly. Complications include arthropathy, arthralgia, osteomyelitis, liver granulomas, granulomatous hepatitis, endocarditis, meningitis and transverse myelitis. Rare severe complications include subacute bacterial endocarditis, orchitis, neuritis (unilateral in 2–10%), neuropathy, cholecystitis and osteomyelitis of the vertebral sacroiliac joint, spondylitis and peripheral reactive arthropathy. Medication includes doxycycline or co-trimoxazole, but steroids, streptomycin, gentamicin and rifampicin have been used. Brucellosis is caused by a Gram-negative, non-spore-forming aerobe coccobacillus that is small, non-motile and non-encapsulated. Four species are known in the human, these being, in order of severity:

answers

1. *Brucella melitensis*
2. *Brucella abortus*
3. *Brucella suis*
4. *Brucella canis*.

143 D

Chlamydia trachomatis is an obligate intracellular parasite. It contains muramic acid in its cell wall and has an independent metabolic activity. It has its own DNA and RNA applications but does not synthesise ATP. The main reservoir is humans and *Chlamydia trachomatis* is susceptible to antibiotics. It causes:

1. Lymphogranuloma venereum
2. Neonatal pneumonitis
3. Non-specific urethritis
4. Endocarditis
5. Pelvic inflammatory disease
6. Trachoma.

This infections usually occurs 5–14 days after delivery and presents with marked bilateral purulent conjunctivitis and respiratory difficulty. It may also be associated with middle ear effusion and infection, and afebrile pneumonia in infancy. On examination, there is marked subcostal and intercostal recession with bilateral crackles and wheeze, and the crusted secretions of purulent conjunctivitis are noticed. Investigations confirm polycythaemia, raised levels of immunoglobulins IgG, IgA and IgM and a high eosinophil count; a nasopharyngeal aspirate may be positive for the parasite. The nasal discharge may be stained with Giemsa to confirm the organism, and immunofluorescence and conjunctival scrapings are often used for diagnosis. Treatment may include erythromycin (children), tetracycline (adults), humidified oxygen, nasogastric feeds and nebulisers.

144 D

Mumps is caused by an RNA paramyxovirus. It is often associated with worldwide endemic episodes that increase during the winter and springtime. Mumps is spread by droplets, and the virus replicates within the epithelial respiratory cells. The virus travels to the parotid gland and disseminates within the central nervous system. It has a 14- to 21-day incubation period from the onset of the parotid swelling to complete resolution. Clinically, the child may present with a 3- to 4-day history of a high fever, malaise, and parotitis that is unilateral in 25% of cases and involves the salivary submandibular glands in 10%. Parotitis is uncomfortable and is due to a red and swollen ostium of Stensen's duct. On examination, the swollen parotid glands are involved in 65% of cases and the submandibular glands in 10%. It is the most common cause of viral meningitis in teenagers in the UK. It may be associated with unilateral deafness in 1/20000 and unilateral orchitis. Other complications include meningoencephalitis (50%), unilateral deafness (10%), pancreatitis, oophoritis, mastitis, unilateral orchitis (20–30% of adults, <5% in children), transverse myelitis, myocarditis and a facial nerve palsy. Medication includes vaccination with MMR (measles, mumps, rubella), but this vaccine may cause a secondary orchitis if not already suffered. Vaccination does not prevent infection after exposure. Immunoglobulin does not ameliorate the disease and has no value. Immunity derived from the vaccine lasts for 20 years, and pregnancy must be avoided for 3 months after the vaccination.

145 C

Glandular fever (infectious mononucleosis) has an incubation period of 10–50 days and is caused by Epstein–Barr virus-infected B cells causing a polyclonal activation of atypical T cells, which causes immortalisation. Clinically, the children present with a high fever and chronic fatigue, often with associated pharyngitis with severe upper airway obstruction. There may be marked lymphadenopathy, and a maculopapular rash with ampicillin. The maculopapular rash may occasionally be haemorrhagic and urticarial in nature but not vesicular. Palatal petechiae may be found in 30% of individuals and may also be seen in other diseases, but are not diagnostic. Jaundice, hepatomegaly and splenomegaly may be found in 50% of cases. Hepatitis is commonly associated in 10–15%. Haematuria may be found on urinalysis. Investigations show an atypical lymphocytosis with mild thrombocytopenia. There is raised aspartate and aminotransaminases, with a raised alkaline phosphatase level.

An atypical lymphocytosis is associated with Epstein–Barr virus, cytomegalovirus, toxoplasmosis, tuberculosis, mumps and malarial infections. It may also be associated with Burkitt's lymphoma, B-cell driven lymphoma, and nasopharyngeal carcinoma in adults. Complications include pneumonitis, pericarditis, upper airway obstruction, seventh cranial nerve palsy, Guillain–Barré syndrome, aseptic meningitis, transverse myelitis, polyneuropathy, nephritis, agranulocytosis and conduction defects.

The Paul–Bunnell test is a circulating heterophile antibody test and may be negative in 50% of paediatric infections. It may be non-specific in 30% in the first week and 90% in the third week. It works by showing the lack of agglutination to both sheep and horse erythrocytes. It may cause a false-positive Wassermann reaction due to polyclonal stimulation.

answers

Extended Matching Answer

146 Theme: Antibiotic actions

1   **C – Cephalosporins**
     D – Isoniazid
     E – Penicillin
     G – Co-trimoxazole
     J – Rifampicin

2   **A – Tetracycline**
     F – Erythromycin
     H – Sulphonamide
     I – Ethambutol

3   **B – Griseofulvin**

The following drugs cause a bactericidal effect: penicillin, cephalosporins, aminoglycosides, co-trimoxazole, rifampicin, isoniazid and pyrazinamide. The following have a bacteriostatic effect: ethambutol, sulphonamides, trimethoprim, erythromycin, chloramphenicol, tetracyclines, vancomycin and clindomycin.

Metabolism

Multiple True/False Answers

147 ABD

X-linked adrenoleukodystrophy has an incidence 1/20 000–50 000 with different phenotypes. It presents in childhood, commonly between 4 and 8 years of age, with progressive intellectual deterioration, seizures, nystagmus, vision and hearing impairment, behavioural and memory disturbance, and progressive neurological decline. Bone marrow transplantation in the early stages of the disease will arrest further progression. It is due to defects of a peroxisomal membrane ATP-binding cassette transporter, associated with elevated levels of very long-chain fatty acids.

148 E

The key features of Refsum's disease are cerebellar ataxia, mixed polyneuropathy and retinitis pigmentosa; the onset is slowly progressive, with 40% of cases presenting before 10 years of age. The sensorimotor polyneuropathy often begins in the distal lower extremities and becomes central with time. Other features include sensorineural hearing loss, cardiac conduction defects and cardiomyopathy, the latter being the commonest cause of death in untreated patients.

The metabolic cause is phytanol coenyzme A hydroxylase deficiency, which leads to an increase in phytanic acid level. The treatment is a dietary restriction of phytanic acid, and plasmapheresis has been used in individuals with very high levels.

Best of Five Answer

149 B

Galactose-1-phosphate uridyl transferase deficiency can present with failure to thrive, sepsis or both. Babies may have hypoglycaemia, diarrhoea and vomiting following an exposure to galactose in the diet. Hepatic dysfunction arises as a consequence of the accumulation of galactose-1-phosphate in the liver; this can lead to hepatosplenomegaly, with abnormal liver function tests and elevated bilirubin levels. Postprandial hypoglycaemia seems to be due to an inhibition of phosphoglucomutase by galactose-1-phosphate, thereby causing inhibition of glycogenolysis.

Red cell assay can be used to measure the function of galactose-1-phosphate uridyl transferase. Dietary elimination prevents further manifestations of the disease. It can be screened for at birth.

Neonatology

Multiple True/False Answers

150 E

Corticosteroids administered for an anticipated premature delivery are associated with a decreased incidence of intraventricular haemorrhage, hyaline membrane disease and neonatal mortality. Combining them with thyrotrophin does not alter the neonatal outcome, although there is an increased incidence of maternal side-effects.

151 ABCDE

Nuchal thickness is the measurement of the subcutaneous tissue over the cervical spine as seen on an ultrasound scan at 11–14 weeks' gestation. It acts as a marker for trisomy 21, 18 and 13. Increased nuchal thickness is associated with other sex chromosome abnormalities and cardiac defects, among other conditions. The associated cardiac lesions include hypoplastic left heart, transposition of the great arteries, coarctation of the aorta, aortic stenosis, ventricular septal defect, endocardial cushion defect and other complex cardiac lesions.

152 None is true

The stillbirth rate is the number of stillbirths per year. The perinatal mortality rate is the number of deaths due to stillbirths in the early neonatal period, that is, those deaths occurring in the first week after delivery. The infant mortality rate is the number of deaths from delivery up to the end of the first year, per yearly period.

Small for gestational age is defined as less than the 10th centile for the matched gestational age; conversely, large for gestational age is greater than the 90th centile for age. Low birthweight is under 2.5 kg, very low birthweight is less than 1.5 kg, and extremely low birthweight is under 1 kg.

answers

153 ABCDE

Other causes include the constitutionally large baby of a large mother, the infant of a diabetic mother, Beckwith–Wiedemann's, Marshall and Weaver syndromes.

154 None is true

There are no randomised controlled trials for any of these procedures; only observational studies exist.

Best of Five Answers

155 D

Risk factors for congenital dislocation of the hip include a positive family history in 20% of cases, female gender (female:male = 6:1), breech delivery in 30%, spina bifida but not spina occulta, being the first born (1 in 100), having a first-degree relative with the condition (1 in 15) and oligohydramnios. It is also more common in the left hip than the right. There is a reduced incidence in premature infants owing to the absence of joint-relaxing maternal hormones. Congenital dislocation of the hip is not associated with caesarean section. Investigations should include a hip ultrasound scan as a diagnosis cannot be made reliably by radiography.

156 A

Hydrops fetalis is the term given to a severe infection found in fetuses and newborns with: (a) a high output cardiac failure, (b) an increase in fluid retention, and (c) acute or chronic anaemia (usually <12 g/dl). The recognised causes of hydrops fetalis include fetomaternal haemorrhage, paroxysmal superventricular tachycardia, Turner's syndrome (lymphoedema), intrauterine and congenital infections (cytomegalovirus, toxoplasmosis, parvovirus, *Treponema pallidum* infection, myocarditis, placental chorioangioma). The scenario given suggests a fetomaternal haemorrhage at 35 + 2 weeks' gestation. *Listeria monocytogenes* and group B haemolytic streptococci are not associated with hydrops fetalis.

157 D

Intrauterine growth retardation is associated with smoking in pregnancy, lower socioeconomic class, malnutrition in pregnancy, alcohol abuse, chromosomal abnormalities, congenital infections and drugs. Features include hypothermia, thermal instability, polycythaemia (secondary to chronic hypoxia or birth asphyxia), hypoglycaemia (secondary to reduced

glycogen stores and impaired glucogenesis), neutropenia, thrombocytopenia and necrotising enterocolitis. The following are not associated with intrauterine growth retardation: anaemia, respiratory distress syndrome (respiratory distress syndrome offers protection due to stress factor) and a loss of birth weight of 10%, which may be normal in a full-term infant who is having feeding difficulties.

158

1　**B – Beckwith–Wiedemann syndrome**

2　**C – Intravenous glucocorticoids and diazoxide**

3　**B – Nephroblastoma**

Neonatal hypoglycaemia is very common in all neonatal units. A blood sugar level <2.6 mmol/l is important to recognise as cerebral activity is affected when the sugar level is this low. Many cases may be asymptomatic so it is essential that neonates and infants in the high-risk categories are appropriately screened to prevent prolonged hypoglycaemia, which may cause a poor neurodevelopmental outcome. Hypoglycaemia in neonates is seen in the following conditions and circumstances:

- prematurity
- intrauterine growth retardation
- intrapartum asphyxia
- hyperthermia
- starvation or poor feeding
- cold stress
- hyaline membrane disease
- polycythaemia
- rhesus blood group incompatibility
- infections.

Metabolic hyperinsulinism and hypoglycaemia may present in older children during an episode of illness or starvation. Endocrine causes usually present in infancy. Causes of hyperinsulinism include:

- infant of an insulin-dependent diabetic mother
- nesidioblastosis
- Beckwith–Wiedemann syndrome
- severe haemolytic disease of the newborn
- islet cell adenoma
- islet cell dysregulation syndrome.

Other rarer causes include hypoxic-ischaemic encephalopathy, septo-optic dysplasia, maternal drug abuse and aminoacidopathies. Treatment options include early and frequent feeds, intravenous dextrose infusions, 3 ml/kg of 10% dextrose in severe cases and intramuscular glucagon only

answers

if there is no access (30–100 µg/kg); in resistant cases 12.5–15.0% dextrose, intravenous glucagon and intravenous glucocorticoids have been used.

Extended Matching Answer

159 Theme: Neonatal seizures

1 **D – Benign familial neonatal convulsions**

2 **G – DiGeorge syndrome**

3 **H – Drug withdrawal**

There is an incidence of 6 in 1000 infants having neonatal seizures. The aetiology of neonatal seizures is vast. Seizures within the first week of life may be due to stroke, Group B haemolytic *Streptococcus*, hypomagnesaemia, maternal opiate addiction, hypoxic-ischaemia encephalopathy (60%), birth asphyxia (50%), intraventricular haemorrhage (15–20%), dural haematoma within 24 hours of delivery, grade IV periventricular haemorrhage, subarachnoid haemorrhage, fifth-day fits and benign familial neonatal convulsions. Other causes include idiopathic (30%), meningitis or encephalitis (20%), hypoglycaemia (10%), hypocalcaemia, hyponatraemia, hypernatraemia, congenital malformations and inborn errors of metabolism, including vitamin B6 pyridoxine deficiency, kernicterus and maple syrup urine disease.

Drug withdrawal is becoming increasingly common, and associated substance abuse includes narcotics, heroin and methadone. Maternal medication, including antituberculous drugs and isoniazid, should be used with caution. Hypophenylalanaemia and maternal antiepileptic treatment do not cause seizures within the first week of life. Hypercalcaemia and hyperkalaemia do not cause neonatal seizures. Wilson's disease, lead poisoning, hypercalcaemic tetany, hyperphosphataemia and hypomagnesaemia cause seizures outside the neonatal period.

Nephrology

Multiple True/False Answers

160 BCDE

Fanconi's syndrome is due to a generalised disorder of proximal tubular reabsorption, thus leading to glycosuria, phosphaturia, hyper-aminoaciduria, calciuria and a loss of bicarbonate into the urine. Sodium reabsorption is also in impaired, compensatory mechanisms leading to potassium and hydrogen ion loss. Salt and water loss cause polyuria, failure to thrive and polydipsia. The bicarbonate loss leads to metabolic acidosis.

The following inborn errors of metabolism are associated with Fanconi's syndrome:

- Nephropathic cystinosis
- Galactosaemia
- Tyrosinaemia
- Wilson's disease
- Fructose intolerance.

The toxic effects of drugs such as tetracycline can cause Fanconi's syndrome, as can heavy metals such as lead, cadmium, thallium and mercury.

161 CDE

Posterior urethral valves occur only in males, affecting 1/12 000 pregnancies. They may be detected by antenatal ultrasound scanning. The obstruction to outflow causes back-pressure on the kidneys even with in utero intervention using vesicoamniotic shunts because of oligohydramnios and pulmonary hyoplasia, leading to many fetuses dying before birth. There is a spectrum of severity of obstruction, which can lead to renal failure in infancy.

answers

162 ABCE

Most cases are detected in utero as the kidneys are enlarged and echogenic; there may be oligohydramnios and pulmonary hypoplasia, which may cause death in utero or shortly after birth. Survivors may have renal hypertension, which may be seen in the first month of life, older children going on to develop portal hypertension. The liver may be normal or enlarged with intrahepatic dilatation.

The perinatal mortality rate is 30–50%. For those beyond the neonatal period, the survival rate is 80–95% due to dialysis, transplantation and surgical intervention where appropriate.

163 ABCDE

Bacterial and viral infections are associated with haematuria. Other causes include glomerular diseases; renal calculi; anatomical abnormalities, for example pelviureteric junction obstruction, polycystic kidneys; renal malignancy; vascular problems such as arteritis, infarction and thrombosis; haematological disorders, for example clotting disorders and sickle cell disease; drugs, such as haematuria from a haemorrhagic cystitis.

164 E

The first four are post-renal causes of renal failure, another example of which is pelviureteric junction obstruction.

Causes of renal failure can be vascular, glomerular or tubular in origin.

- Vascular examples are renal vein thrombosis, haemolytic–uraemic syndrome and arterial occlusion.
- Any cause of glomerular disease can be responsible.
- Tubular dysfunction can be caused by nephrotoxins, for example drugs such as gentamicin, myoglobulinuria, haemoglobinuria and acute interstitial nephritis.

165 ABCDE

Screening for urinary tract infection should always be included in the investigations for enuresis. Detrusor instability is characterized by daytime frequency, urgency and incontinence throughout the day. Neuropathic bladder also shows daytime wetting, which may be associated with soiling and an abnormal gait or abnormal lower extremities; the bladder may also be palpable. Diabetes mellitus is revealed by polyuria, weight loss and thirst. Ectopic ureters are associated with dribbling that continues after voiding.

Best of Five Answer

166 E

Alport's syndrome is otherwise known as childhood hereditary nephritis. It is transmitted through the maternal linkage and displays variable penetrance. It shows X-linked dominance and autosomal dominance with a high mutation rate. It is expressed in males but may also be expressed in females to a lesser degree. This disorder may be silent during childhood and present in adolescence with asymptomatic haematuria and proteinuria. The glomerulus and the basement of the cochlear nerve have similar pathological defects, with weakness of the basement membrane: a defect in the α5 type 4 collagen basement membrane chainlinked to the gene col4a5. This is the same defect as occurs in Goodpasture's syndrome. The antigen recognised by the Goodpasture's antibody, which resides in the α3 chain of type 4 collagen, is usually **absent**, and therefore the glomeruli do not react with the antiglomerular basement membrane antibodies. These children, if male and severely affected, die from chronic renal failure between 25 and 40 years of age. Females may have a normal life span and suffer only mild hearing loss.

Berger's glomerulonephritis is usually associated with group A haemolytic *Streptococcus*. Pendred's syndrome is often associated with hypothyroidism, and children with Laurence–Moon–Biedl syndrome show a typical dysmorphic appearance. Children with congenital nephrotic syndrome usually present in the first year of life.

167

1   **C – Post-renal failure**

2   **D – Haemolytic–uraemic syndrome**

3   **C – Nephrocalcinosis**

This child was initially suffering from post-renal failure secondary to haemolytic–uraemic syndrome. He subsequently suffered from the complications of nephrocalcinosis and was found to be in chronic renal failure. All other diagnoses given in part 3 present with acute renal failure. Renal failure is thought of in three categories:

- *Pre-renal failure*: In this category there is a decrease in intravascular volume, effective volume depletion and glomerular filtration rate so a highly concentrated urine is excreted. There is an increase in the metabolism of the renin–angiotensin system, aldosterone secretion and sodium reabsorption/potassium excretion in the distal tubules. Sodium levels can be maintained.

answers

- *Intrinsic renal failure*: In this category, acute tubular necrosis is inevitable. The kidney is unable to reabsorb sodium or concentrate urea.
- *Post-renal failure*: In this category the failure is caused by renal obstruction, ie nephrocalcinosis.

Other drugs that may be harmful in the treatment of chronic renal failure include oxytetracyclines (all except doxycycline) as all increase urea production. The sulphonamide component of antibiotics causes interstitial nephritis, and ibuprofen decreases the glomerular filtration rate if the patient has impaired renal function, ie the patient is elderly or is in cardiac failure.

Extended Matching Answers

168 Theme: Urinary discoloration

1   **B – Tetracyclines**

2   **A – Myoglobulinaemia**
     F – Levodopa

3   **I – Rifampicin**

4   **C – Phenolphthalein**
     E – Laxative abuse
     J – Acute intravascular haemolysis

5   **H – Iron**

6   **D – Phenylketonuria**
     G – Isoniazid

Red urine is the result of acute haemolysis, and red blood cells may be noted on microscopy. Brown smoky urine may be due to a disease of the glomerulus, and the cells on microscopy are distorted, small and fragmented. Red cell casts may be seen. Haematuria from the bladder or urethra may show normal cells on microscopy.

Causes of a brown urine include levodopa, methyldopa, myoglobinuria, Alport's syndrome with associated glomerular sclerosis, congenital biliary atresia, bowel disease, acute porphyria (porphobilinogen), porphyria variegata and congenital porphyria. A red urine can arise from rifampicin, dyes, laxative abuse, phenolphthalein, acute intravascular haemolysis, haemoglobinuria (urobilinogen), beetroot, acute intermittent porphyria, *Serratia marcescens*, haematuria associated with hereditary telangiectasia and Wilms' tumour.

Causes of a pink urine include rifampicin, dyes and urates. A yellow urine can result from taking tetracyclines. Causes of a black urine include iron, homogentisic acid and melanotic sarcomas. Causes of blue urine, especially noted in nappies, include idicanuria.

Drugs which show no change in the urinary colour include isoniazid, and disorders with the same effect include phenylketonuria.

169 Theme: Haematuria

1   **B – Benign familial haematuria**
     D – Henoch–Schönlein purpura
     F – Cyclophosphamide therapy
     H – Hereditary telangiectasia
     J – Beetroot ingestion

2   **A – Haemophilia**
     C – Glucose-6-phosphate deficiency
     E – Tumour lysis syndrome
     F – Cyclophosphamide therapy
     I – Familial nephritis

3   **J – Beetroot ingestion**

Haematuria is seen in 2% of normal schoolchildren and presents with microscopic-macroscopic asymptomatic haematuria. The disorders are usually benign. Macroscopic haematuria may settle and become microscopic in nature.

Causes of microscopic haematuria include benign familial haematuria, Henoch–Schönlein purpura, cyclophosphamide therapy, hereditary telangiectasia and beetroot ingestion. Other causes include dysplastic or congenital renal tract abnormalities, hydronephrosis, membranous nephritis, insulin-dependent diabetes mellitus-associated glomerular sclerosis, hypercalciuria secondary to hypercalcaemia, vascular arteritis and vascular vasculitis. Documented causes include acute tubular necrosis, congenital nephritic syndrome, exercise, factitious disease, Williams' syndrome and drugs including ciclosporin, rifampicin and cyclophosphamide.

Causes of macroscopic haematuria include haemophilia, glucose-6-phosphatase deficiency, tumour lysis syndrome, sickle cell disease and familial nephritis. Other causes include urinary tract infections, malaria, schistosomiasis, trauma (falling over the handlebars of a bicycle), IgA nephropathy, glomerular sclerosis, nephrocalcinosis, idiopathic hypercalciuria, nephroblastoma, neuroblastoma, IgA deficiency and Alport's syndrome.

Neurology

Multiple True/False Answers

170 ADE

Half of those children who have an afebrile fit will have another episode. The population risk for a febrile convulsion is between 2.7% and 3.3%.

171 ABCD

Absence seizures are sudden brief periods of unconsciousness, typical seizures showing regular, symmetrical, generalised spike and wave complexes occurring at three cycles per second. About 10% of fits in children with epilepsy are due to typical absence seizures, and if this is the only manifestation, the prognosis is very good.

Affected children may have an alteration in school performance so an educational history involving the main teacher is an important part of the history.

172 ACDE

The list of prenatally determined causes of hydrocephalus includes:

- neural tube defects
- Arnold–Chiari malformation
- hydranencephaly
- achondroplasia
- schizencephaly
- arachnoid cysts
- isolated or sex-linked stenosis of the Sylvian aqueduct
- aneurysm of the vein of Galen
- Hurler's disease
- lissencephaly.

Acquired hydrocephalus has the following causes:

- *Post haemorrhagic* – such as neonatal intraventricular haemorrhage, subarachnoid or subdural haemorrhage.

- *Post meningitic* – toxoplasmosis, mumps, cytomegalovirus, rubella, tuberculosis, toxoplasmosis.
- *Space-occupying lesions* – tumour, clot, cyst, abscess.

Other causes are fungal infection, cysticercosis, sarcoidosis and spinal tumour.

173 ABCDE

Causes of basal calcification are as follows:

- *Endocrine* – hypo/hyperparathyroidism, pseudo and pseudopseudoparathyroidism, hypothyroidism.
- *Congenital and metabolic disease* – mitochondrial encephalopathies, Leigh's encephalopathy, carbon monoxide poisoning, systemic lupus erythematosus, Down's syndrome, tuberous sclerosis, neurofibromatosis.
- *Infection* – toxoplasmosis, cytomegalovirus, subacute sclerosing panencephalitis, congenital rubella, acquired immunedeficiency syndrome.
- *Neoplasms* – craniopharyngioma, radiotherapy or methotrexate treatment for leukaemia.

174 D

Regression associated with seizures is seen in:

- GM2 gangliosidosis
- Gaucher's disease
- Sialidosis type 1
- Batten disease.

Regression without epilepsy is seen in:

- Juvenile Huntington's disease
- Adrenoleukodystrophy
- Metachromatic leukodystrophy
- Subacute sclerosing panencephalitis
- Wilson's disease.

Regression in toddlers with neurological signs is seen with metachromatic leukodystrophy, juvenile Sandhoff's disease, ataxia telangiectasia, Leigh's disease and Niemann–Pick disease type C. Regression in toddlers with autistic features is seen with Rett's syndrome, Angelman syndrome and infantile Batten disease.

answers

175 B

The International Headache Society has the following criteria for migraine without an aura:

- At least five attacks fulfilling the next three headings, without there being any evidence of organic disease.
- A headache of between 4 and 72 hours' duration.
- The headache has two of the following four features:
  - Unilateral
  - Pulsating
  - Worsened by physical exercise
  - Affects daily activities.
- There should be one of the following – photophobia/phonophobia/nausea/vomiting.

The criteria for abdominal migraine include:

- Pain limiting daily activities
- Dullness or soreness
- Periumbilical or poorly localised
- Associated loss of appetite
- Nausea/vomiting
- Pallor
- Attacks of abdominal pain lasting for at least 1 hour; there should be resolution between attacks, which should occur at least twice a year.

Best of Five Answer

176 B

Migraine is very common in women (18%) and men (6%), especially before puberty. There are many forms of migraine including:

- basilar
- classical
- epileptic
- abdominal
- hemiplegic.

Causes of migraine include the oral contraceptive pill, menstruation, diet, stress, anxiety and tiredness; there is often a positive family history. Clinically, the child may present with ataxia, vertigo and travel sickness, but it is more likely that the child will present with severe bilateral and occipital headaches with an associated aura and vomiting. There may be unilateral limb weakness after a severe attack (hemiplegia) or the child may suffer from visual symptoms, tinnitus, ataxia, nystagmus and vertigo (basilar). There may also be associated migranous neuralgia in which the child suffers from unilateral lacrimation. This may occur after a cluster headache and is rare in childhood. In classical pulsating unilateral migraine, there may be associated photophobia, photonia and nausea, and an aura may or may not be present.

An EEG may be undertaken if a fit has been suggested, which will show slow activity during an attack with generalised slow waves, which are focal in nature. This may predict the ischaemic phase of the migraine.

Treatment includes simple analgesics and antiemetics; otherwise, prophylaxis includes pizotifen (a 5-hydroxytyptamine (5HT) antagonist), which is useful in a chronic attack. β-Blockers may help an acute attack. Methysergide may cause obstructive nephropathy but is often used in adulthood. An acute attack may be relieved by 5HT agonists such as sumatriptan, which causes vasoconstriction and is therefore not used in children. Amitriptyline, a tricyclic antidepressant, has also been used. In general pizotifen, an antagonist, is used to vasodilate the vessels and is used in chronic prophylaxis. Sumatriptan is an agonist and causes vasoconstriction; it is used in the acute phase. The differential diagnosis includes porphyria, epilepsy, depression and a subarachnoid haemorrhage.

Extended Matching Answer

177 Theme: Neuromuscular disorders

1 **D – Duchenne muscular dystrophy**

Duchenne muscular dystrophy is found in 1 in 3000 live male births and is X-linked recessive in nature. It is found at the XP21 locus. A total of 75% of cases may be sporadic; 66% of cases are familial, 33% are due to new mutations, and 50% of the mothers are carriers. Carrier status results from lyonisation and not translocation. This disorder is not associated with maternal age. Women may be symptomatic due to random inactivation of one of the X chromosomes and failure to inactivate the maternal X chromosome. Duchenne muscular dystrophy may be found in children who have Turner's syndrome (45XO).

2 **G – Becker's muscular dystrophy**

Becker's muscular dystrophy usually presents between 6 and 16 years of age, and the abnormality is found at the same locus as Duchenne muscular dystrophy (XP21). Both disorders are caused by a mutation of the dystrophin gene. Genetic coding is abnormal in both disorders, but mutation of the dystrophin gene is less likely in Becker's muscular dystrophy. In this condition, there is a decreased level of dystrophin and the dystrophin product, which is functionally more normal. In Duchenne muscular dystrophy, there is no dystrophin present and therefore no functional product.

Neonatal diagnosis may be performed by deletion screening. The dystrophin gene is short, abnormal and non-functional, and has negative immune-labelled protein. In contrast, Becker's muscular dystrophy may have positive immune-labelled dystrophin depending on how abnormal the gene is.

Children with Becker's muscular dystrophy usually have a normal IQ. In children with Duchenne's muscular dystrophy, however, the IQ is lowered by 10–20 points.

3   **H – Polio**

Poliovirus infection is caused by a picorna enterovirus, of which there are three serotypes. Type 1 is the virus mainly responsible for outbreaks of paralytic polio, and type 2 is the strongest immunogen, which gives the highest rate of seroconversion after vaccination. This virus is transmitted by the faecal–oral route, being found in food, water and milk in African countries. The virus enters the gastrointestinal tract and multiplies in the epithelial cells of the Peyer's patches and tonsils. It then spreads through the lymph node system for further multiplication and spread to the bloodstream. The acute febrile illness is thereby initiated, and there is dissemination of the virus to the reticuloendothelial cells, which causes the viraemia.

In the region of 90–95% of asymptomatic patients present with lymphadenopathy, 4–8% with a mild febrile illness and 1–2% with aseptic meningitis; 1% present with classic paralytic polio, which is associated with a painful stiff gait and lower limb paralysis. The virus affects the anterior horn cells of the spinal cord so the legs are more affected than the arms. The cranial nuclei of the brainstem cause bulbar polio, which affects the cells of the motor cortex. Paralysis is less common in children than adults, and a tonsillectomy will increase the incidence of bulbar polio.

The virus can be grown from a stool culture for up to 5 weeks after the onset of illness, and serology is positive if there is a fourfold increase in titre between the acute and convalescence samples. Investigations undertaken usually include a stool sample, which will be inoculated with monkey kidney cells to grow the virus. Pharyngeal washings, lumbar puncture samples and paired serum antibody titres are also taken.

Conduction tests show a delayed response, and an EEG and EMG are normal. Caution should be taken in undertaking a lumbar puncture as this may increase paralysis if the patient is not already paralysed.

Treatment includes bed rest in the acute phase, observation of respiratory and bulbar complications, physiotherapy and, initially, with a raised white cell count, treatment with antibiotics and aciclovir. This disease is a communicable disease and must be reported; in addition, the community must be immunised. The differential diagnosis includes Guillain–Barré syndrome, transverse myelitis, aseptic meningitis, porphyria, peripheral neuropathy and toxin overdose.

Oncology

Multiple True/False Answers

178 DE

The staging for neuroblastoma is as follows:

- *Stage 1*: Localised tumour confined to the area of origin, complete gross excision, without or with microscopic residual disease and identifiable ipsilateral and contralateral lymph nodes that are negative microscopically.
- *Stage 2A*: Unilateral tumour with incomplete gross excision and identifiable ipsilateral and contralateral lymph nodes that are negative microscopically.
- *Stage 2*: Unilateral tumour with complete or incomplete gross excision, with positive ipsilateral regional lymph nodes and identifiable contralateral lymph nodes that are negative microscopically.
- *Stage 3*: Tumour infiltrating across the midline with or without regional lymph node involvement; or unilateral tumour with contralateral regional lymph node involvement; or midline tumour with bilateral regional lymph node involvement.
- *Stage 4*: Dissemination of tumour to distant lymph nodes, bone, bone marrow, liver and/or other organs (except as defined in stage 4S)
- *Stage 4S*: Localised primary tumour as defined for stages 1 and 2 but with dissemination limited to the liver, skin and/or bone marrow.

Amplification of the proto-oncogene *MYCN* is associated with a poorer prognosis, as is deletion of the short arm of chromosome 1 at 1p and gain of the long arm of chromosome 17 at 17q. A good outcome is associated with the high-affinity nerve growth factor TrkA and the low-affinity nerve growth factor. Diploid or tetraploid tumours have a poorer outlook than hyperploid tumours. Infants have a better prognosis overall than older children.

179 DE

The incidence of sacrococcygeal tumours in the UK is 1/35 000, girls being more commonly affected than boys. Two-thirds of the tumours are benign, 39% are malignant and 5–10% are immature. The most common site is localised to the buttocks; fewer have intrapelvic or intraabdominal extension. Surgical removal is mandatory, as is the measurement of alphafetoprotein, human chorionic gonadotrophin and urinary catecholamines to ensure that a pelvic neuroblastoma is excluded. Pulmonary metastases must also be excluded.

Best of Five Answers

180 C

Hodgkin's disease has two peak age groups – 15–25 years and 55–75 years old. It shows human leukocyte antigen (HLA) association and familial clustering. The disease presents as a fluctuating course with an 80% 5-year survival rate. It is more common in men than women.

The clinical presentation may include painless cervical lymphadenopathy, fever, sweating, pruritis, bone pain and hepatosplenomegaly. These 'B' symptoms are not common and may present in 25–35% in early diagnosis. They include fever >38°C, drenching night sweats, an unexplained weight loss of >10%, pruritis, alcohol-induced pain (1–10%) and a lymphocyte count <1.5 × 10^9 cells/l. Common sites of metastasis include the lymph nodes, bone, bone marrow and liver.

Methods of staging include the Ann Arbor staging system, lymph node biopsy and histology. Lymphocyte-predominant Hodgkin's disease displays the best prognosis, with few Reed–Sternberg cells, whereas lymphocyte-depleted disease, with mostly Reed–Sternberg cells present, has the worst prognosis. Hepatocellular carcinoma presents in adult life due to persistent damage of hepatitis B surface antigen (HBsAg) positivity. Aspergilloma is more likely to be found in the immunocompromised host. Ibuprofen does not cause an autoimmune haemolytic anaemia.

181 C

AML is a disorder of maturation of the haematological precursors. It is less common than ALL (the ALL:AML ratio being 80:20). AML is, however, more common than CML in children. AML represents 20% of all leukaemias. There is an equal incident ratio between men and women. The prognosis if affected by the patient's age, and AML has a 5-year

answers

survival rate of 40–50%. There are a few conditions that are associated with a high risk of developing AML, such as Franconi's anaemia, Bloom's syndrome, Down's syndrome and immunosuppression.

AML is classified according to the FAB classification. Children with the M3 FAB classification (promyelocytic – APML) often present with disseminated intravascular coagulation, and patients are treated with retinoic acid receptase (RAR) prior to induction of remission in M3. The bleeding is caused by a procoagulant material present in the blasts. If this is present, early mortality may occur. ATRA decreases this early mortality by enabling cells to differentiate beyond the promyelocytic state. Children may present with gum hypertrophy, gum bleeding, fever, bruising, rectal infiltration and ulceration, and skin involvement. Complications include bleeding and fatal cerebral haemorrhage. Myeloblastic chloromas are solid deposits of AML around the orbits, spinal cord and cranium, and may cause proptosis.

Multiple True/False Questions

182 ABE

Optic atrophy secondary to a neoplasm as well as primary optic atrophy can be a cause, as is unilateral cataract and VIth cranial nerve dysfunction.

183 ABCDE

Other causes include neurometabolic disorders such as Leigh's disease, organic acidaemia, urea cycle disorders and aminoacidaemias.

Best of Five Answer

184 E

This is a classical presentation of uveitis. A flare is seen due to keratic deposits on the corneal endothelium and a reflection from scattered light from a beam shone into the eye. Erythema results from inflammatory cells in the aqueous humour and within the uveal tract. Fibrous exudates on the lens surface cause the presence of a hypopyon. Chronic changes include glaucoma, cataract formation and retinal damage.

Extended Matching Answers

185 Theme: Ophthalmoscopy
1   **B – Congenital rubella**
     E – Insulin-dependent diabetes mellitus
     G – Herpes simplex infection
     J – Hurler's syndrome

answers

2   **A – Trauma to the cornea**
     C – Glaucoma
     D – TORCH infections
     I – Chronic keratitis

3   **F – Hunter's syndrome**

Corneal clouding is characteristic of Hurler's syndrome and is often termed corneal opacification, although this is not necessarily the correct terminology. The majority of those with mucopolysaccharidoses (excluding Hunter's syndrome) will develop corneal changes within 2 years. Tuberous sclerosis presents with phakomatas and tubers of the retina. Osteogenesis imperfecta presents with blue sclerae, and galactosaemia with cataracts. Both Marfan's syndrome and homocystinuria present with ectopia lentis.

186 Theme: Papillary signs

1   **C – Barbiturate usage**
     D – Metabolic conditions
     H – Opiate usage

2   **A – Severe hypoxia**
     B – Inner brain damage
     C – Barbiturate usage
     G – Post-seizure activity
     J – Hypothermia

3   **F – Tentorial herniation**

A fixed pinpoint pupil is seen in early barbiturate usage, whereas a fixed dilated pupil is a late presenting sign. Small reactive pupils are seen in metabolic conditions and medullary lesions. Fixed mid-sized pupils are seen in midbrain lesions.

187 Theme: Uveitis

1   **E – Toxocariasis**
     F – Toxoplasmosis

Infectious causes of uveitis include toxoplasmosis, tuberculosis, toxocariasis, tertiary syphilis, human immunodeficiency virus, herpes simplex virus, cytomegalovirus, Epstein–Barr virus and meningococcal disease.

2   **H – Sarcoidosis**
     I – Behçet's disease

Musculoskeletal diseases associated with uveitis include sarcoidosis, seronegative arthritis and Behçet's disease.

3   **A – Crohn's disease**
     B – Whipple's disease

Inflammatory diseases commonly associated with uveitis include Crohn's disease, and Whipple's disease and *rarely* ulcerative colitis. Other causes of uveitis include sympathetic uveitis in the eye contralateral to the one associated with trauma, multiple sclerosis and Vogt-Koyanagi-Harada syndrome. Treatment options include treatment of the underlying disease, topical agents (local and systemic steroids), mydriatics and an eye patch.

188 Theme: Visual field disorders

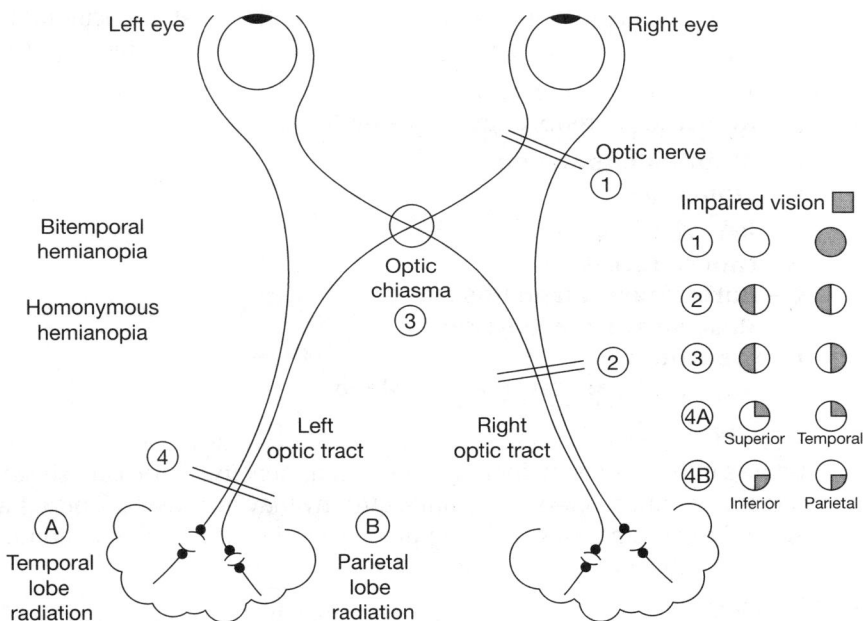

Left eye   Right eye

Optic nerve
①

Impaired vision ▨

Bitemporal
hemianopia
                          Optic
                          chiasma
Homonymous   ③
hemianopia

                                              ②

              Left   Right
④   optic tract   optic tract

Ⓐ   Ⓑ
Temporal   Parietal
lobe   lobe
radiation   radiation

① ◯ ⬤
② ◑ ◐
③ ◑ ◐
④A ◖Superior ◖Temporal
④B ◗Inferior ◗Parietal

1   **D – Bitemporal hemianopia**
     E – Bitemporal superior quadrantanopia

2   **D – Bitemporal hemianopia**
     F – Bitemporal inferior quadrantanopia

These scenarios describe optic chiasm dysfunction. The patient is only able to see objects directly in front of their face, and peripheral lateral vision is impaired. She suffers from bitemporal superior quadrantanopia due to compression of the chiasm from below (ie the pituitary). He suffers from compression from above (ie the suprasellar region) which

299

answers

results in an inferior quadrantanopia. Causes include acromegaly, optic glioma, pituitary adenoma, prolactinoma, craniopharyngioma, chordomas and hysterical phenomena. Cushing's disease causes microadenomata that are too small to cause an effect.

3   **A – Optic nerve dysfunction**

Optic nerve dysfunction may present as either unilateral or bilateral blindness. It presents with impaired visual acuity, poor colour vision and an afferent pupil defect. If the optic nerve is associated with a demyelinating disease (ie multiple sclerosis), a papillitis may occur, and this may be associated with raised ultracranial pressure, optic atrophy, optic disc oedema and retinal tumour. Optic nerve dysfunction may be seen in Weber's syndrome, which presents with ipsilateral oculomotor nerve palsy, contralateral hemiplegia and a paralysis of upward gaze.

189 Theme: Tunnel vision and papilloedema

1   **C – Retinitis pigmentosa**
     F – Glaucoma
     J – Optic atrophy

2   **A – Papilloedema**
     B – Retinal vein thromboses
     E – Malignant hypertension
     F – Glaucoma
     H – Subdural haematoma and bleed

3   **A – Papilloedema**

Causes of tunnel vision include retinitis pigmentosa, choroidoretinitis, papilloedema and glaucoma. Optic atrophy may be an aetiological factor secondary to tabes dorsalis, migraine, hysteria, syphilis and bilateral lesions of the anterior calcarine sulcus.

Causes of papilloedema are many. They may be broken down into systems (Table 13).

Neurological	**Endocrinological**
Raised intracranial pressure	Hypoparathyroidism
Hydrocephalus	Hypocalcaemia
Space-occupying lesion	Hyperthyroidism + exophthalmos
Subdural haematoma	
Abscess of the brain	**Infectious**
	Tuberculous meningitis
Ophthalmological	
Retinal vein thrombosis	**Pharmacological**
Papillitis	Systemic corticosteroid treatment
	Lead toxicity
Cardiovascular	Vitamin A toxicity
Malignant hypertension	
Benign hypertension	**Oncological**
	Posterior fossa tumour
Respiratory	Lymphoma
Carbon dioxide retention	

Table 13: Causes of papilloedema

Severe myopia and scotoma do not cause papilloedema. Papilloedema may itself cause tunnel vision.

Psychiatry

Multiple True/False Answers

190 BCDE

Child abuse does not recognise social status, ethnic origin or religious persuasion. The following have been identified as risk factors for physical abuse:

- product of an unwanted pregnancy
- low birthweight
- mental or physical handicap
- incessant crying or sleeplessness.

Parental features are:

- single-parent family with poor support – low self-esteem in the parent(s)
- unrealistic expectations and inconsistent discipline or punishment as a means of discipline.

Social circumstances identified as risk factors include domestic friction, a large family, low income and stresses such as a housing crisis.

191 None is true

The values in Table 14 apply to 4-year-old children.

Behavioural problem	%
Poor appetite	20
Difficulty settling at night	15
Overactive and restless	13
Poor concentration	6
Temper	6
Poor relationships with peers	6
Poor relationships with siblings	15
Regular day wetting	8
Regular bed-wetting	19
Regular soiling	3

Table 14: Frequency of behavioural problems in 4-year-olds

192 E

The prevalence of autism in childhood is between 4 and 20/100 000, boys being affected three times more often than girls. Social interaction, lack of eye contact and facial expression, and not taking part in play are common features – it is, however, difficult to be certain about the diagnosis before 2 years of age. Language is delayed and associated with echolalia, poor comprehension and using the third person in place of 'I'. Ritualistic and compulsive behaviour is frequent. IQ scores of 100 are seen in only 5% of children, whereas 70% lie much below this figure.

193 CE

The origin of CFS is as yet unclear; it is suggested that this may be an umbrella term under which may lie different conditions with different aetiologies. The two clinical features required to satisfy the definition of the Centers for Disease Control and Prevention are:

- debilitating fatigue reducing activity to less than 50% of the patient's premorbid activity for at least 6 months
- symptoms not explicable by a medical or psychiatric disorder.

Non-psychotic depression does not exclude CFS.

Four out of the eight following symptom criteria must be present:

- sleep disturbance
- arthralgia
- cervical or axillary lymphadenopathy that is painful
- myalgia
- sore throat
- headaches
- generalised tiredness after the usual level of activity
- neuropsychological features such as lack of concentration and lethargy.

194

1 **D – A Connors' Teachers Rating School Questionnaire**
2 **D – Attention deficit hyperactivity disorder (ADHD)**
3 **C – Methylphenidate hydrochloride**

This child has ADHD. ADHD may be caused by hereditary, emotional, environmental or frontal lobe changes. It is found in 1 in 200 children in the UK, with a prevalence rate of 1–2%. It is more common in boys (3:1 ratio of boys:girls), and one in ten boys in the UK are on methylphenidate hydrochloride. The peak incidence is in the first decade of life. There appears to be a strong hereditary component and a history of limited social function and learning and developmental delay.

answers

The *International Classification of Diseases* (ICD) 10 and the *Diagnostic and Statistical Manual of Mental Disorders* (DSM) IV criteria appear to differ. Overall, three main features exist. These include overactivity, inattention and impulsiveness. Disorders suggested as being linked to ADHD include normal variant of difficult behaviour, conduct disorders, school expulsion, multiple accidents, temporal lobe epilepsy, large families, social deprivation, isolated children and developmental syndromes such as Fragile X syndrome, autistic spectrum disorder and speech and language delay. ADHD may also be found in children with a normal brain.

In general, a normal child with hyperactivity and inattention should not be commenced on a food-exclusion diet or high-dose vitamins. They should not be routinely commenced on methylphenidate hydrochloride either. However, they should be referred to a speech and language therapist if speech delay is noted. Children with ADHD should be referred to a child development centre for the completion of a Connors' Teachers Rating Scale Questionnaire, and their activities and their inattention, both at home and in school, should often be assessed. Family circumstances and parenting skills may need to be addressed.

Treatment options include behaviour modification programmes and stimulant medication, including dexamphetamine and methylphenidate hydrochloride. Side-effects include insomnia, anorexia, abdominal pain, headache, reversible growth inhibition, depression, psychoses, facial tics and seizures. Barbiturates (phenobarbitone) must not be given as they may induce hyperactivity.

195

1   **C – Munchausen by proxy**

2   **A – Poisoning**

3   **E – All of the above**

All five items listed here are definite clues to Munchausen by proxy. Independently, they may explain any number of clinical diseases, but the occurrence of all five together, as in the above case, is highly suspicious of Munchausen by proxy.

Munchausen by proxy is a factitious disease of childhood. The perpetrator is often the child's chief carer, more often the mother. The carer may have a medical background and may be suffering from depression. There is no association with drug misuse. The carer often appears unconcerned but seems to interfere with all investigations. Known associations include repeated loss of consciousness, seizures (but not a history of seizures), hypernatraemia and hypoglycaemia. Clinical presentation may often be loss of consciousness, drowsiness, asystole, fever, dehydration, vomiting, hypoglycaemia, haematuria, haematemesis, diarrhoea, failure to thrive or trauma with no corresponding history. Aetiological causes include poisoning (salt), drug ingestion/injection (insulin), apnoea by suffocation (pillow), sexual abuse and physical injury (fractures).

Munchausen by proxy is not the same as malingering, in which patients have insight and there is often a recognisable environmental goal of producing symptoms beyond assuming the sick role. Munchausen by proxy is not somatisation as there is no insight and it is characterised by multiple physical complaints. It is not hysterical conversion disorder either, as there is no insight and such a disorder (ie conversion) is characterised by physical, often neurological, symptoms that produce primary and secondary gain but not consciously produced by the patient.

Extended Matching Questions

196 Theme: Behaviour disorders

a) 1 Description A – Bulimia nervosa;
Description B – Anorexia nervosa;
Description C – Bulimia nervosa, Anorexia nervosa and
Behaviour disorder;
Description D – Behaviour disorder;
Description E – Bulimia nervosa;
Description F – Anorexia nervosa;
Description G – Anorexia nervosa;
Description H – Bulimia nervosa and anorexia nervosa;
Description I – Bulimia nervosa and anorexia nervosa

b) 1 Diagnosis C – Bulimia nervosa
2 Diagnosis E – Anorexia nervosa
3 Diagnosis A – Behaviour disorder

Bulimia nervosa is the most common chronic physiological eating disorder, with a prevalence of 1% and an age presentation between 17 and 18 years of age. There is a predominance in girls, with only 10% of cases presenting in boys. The *International Classification of Diseases* (ICD) 10 criteria state that:

(1) Bulimia nervosa is a preoccupation with eating that causes overeating.
(2) The resultant anxiety is counteracted by the vomiting and purging of food substances.
(3) The fear of fatness and a distorted body image results.

Binge eating is pathognomonic of bulimia nervosa and is not a sign of recovery. Approximately 25% of bulimia nervosa patients are overweight

answers

prior to their disease, whereas 40% of anorexia nervosa patients are overweight beforehand. Sufferers may abuse laxatives, diuretics and stimulants. Amenorrhoea is not required for diagnosis. Clubbing is a late sign. Psychological thoughts include fear of fatness; concealed eating leads to guilt and depression; and meticulous behaviour, as opposed to a neglected appearance, is noted. Associated disorders include impulsive control disorders (drug and alcohol abuse), chaotic families, co-morbid depression and previous child sexual abuse. The prognosis is better than that for anorexia nervosa, with a 50–70% remission rate. Severe vomiting may lead to aspiration and finally death.

Behavioural disorders are increased in children whose family has associated:

- maternal depression
- emotional neglect
- physical and sexual abuse
- a full-time working mother
- a sibling with cystic fibrosis
- a child resident in a residential home.

The ICD10 of emotional disorders consists of: (1) separation anxiety, (2) phobic anxiety, (3) social anxiety and (4) sibling rivalry.

Emotional disorders occur when a child's emotions and behaviour are out of proportion to the expected reaction or may be inappropriate for the child's age. This may be pathological, and these disorders are increased in females, smaller families and where there is a history of depression or anxiety in the family. Emotional disorders are NOT affective disorders, which are more common in the adult population and may cause an increase in depression in the sufferers' children. Emotional disorders are more common in females (2:1), and are seen in social class I societies. Statistically, 60% show unipolar depression and 1% bipolar depression, 1 in 5 require treatment, 1 in 50 require intermittent hospitalisation, and 1 in 200 commit suicide.

197 Theme: Learning difficulty

1 **C – Depression**
   G – Bullying
   J – Child sexual abuse

2 **B – Language delay**
   E – Conduct disorder
   I – Attention deficit hyperactivity disorder (ADHD)

3 **A – Hypothyroidism**
   D – Huntington's chorea

F – Insulinoma
H – Vitamin B12 deficiency

Two per cent of all children have an IQ of <50, while 3–4/1000 have an IQ of 50–70. A total of 25% of learning disability results from genetic inheritance and 25% from environmental factors. There is an increased risk (5- to 6-fold) associated with a psychological disorder. Psychological problems occur in 30% of all cases of moderate learning difficulties and 50% of all those with severe learning difficulties; 36% may have associated epilepsy, but epileptic children have normal intelligence.

Educational underachievement may be found in:

- language disorders
- depression
- deafness
- boredom
- visual problems
- bullying
- reading disorders
- poor teaching
- lack of wider skills
- child sexual abuse
- anti-educational family
- substance abuse.

Specific reading disorders are found in 6% of children, 50% of whom may have an associated psychological disorder. Reading disorders are associated with the following:

- Boys
- Right and left disorientation
- Clumsiness
- Language delay
- Family history
- ADHD
- Conduct disorders.

Intellectual deterioration may be reversible or irreversible and have the following aetiological factors:

- *Reversible*: subdural haemorrhage, hypothyroidism, vitamin B12 deficiency.
- *Irreversible*: Huntington's chorea, insulinoma, chronic alcoholism, general paresis of the insane due to syphilis.

Disorders associated with a low IQ are:

- conduct disorders
- enuresis

answers

- emotional disorders
- encopresis
- school refusal and truancy
- psychoses
- ADHD
- depression
- autism.

198 Theme: Odd behaviour

1   **C – Obsessional neuroses**

2   **B – Diarrhoea**
      D – Dry mouth
      H – Palpitations and sweating
      J – Failure of erection

3   **A – Paraesthesia**
      D – Dry mouth
      E – Dizziness
      G – Panic attacks
      I – Faintness

4   **C – Neck pain**
      F – Tension headache

This boy suffers from obsessive-compulsive disorder (OCD). This is a neurotic illness in which the patient has good insight into the illness. The degree of anxiety is out of proportion to the stress experienced. There is a 3:1 incidence of boys:girls. The obsessions may be recurrent, persistent ideas and thoughts/images (ruminations – repetitive internal arguments) that are inconclusive. The compulsions are impulses to carry out an activity that is non-aggressive. It may be ritualistic and may be triggered by the original obsessional thought. There is no subjective awareness of the hyperventilation. There is a well-recognised association between OCD and depression, occurring in 30% of cases; 25% may develop pre-morbid depression during the illness. A family history of neuroses or of a progression to schizophrenia is not associated with OCD. The overall prognosis is excellent.

The clinical presentation includes impaired concentration, poor memory, disturbed sleep, irritability, restlessness, fearful anticipation, tetany, tachycardia, paraesthesia of the extremities and difficulty in focusing the vision.

The physical symptoms result from autonomic overactivity, hyperventilation, increased smooth muscle tone and panic attacks. Medical management includes reassurance, psychotherapy and benzodiazepines, β-blockers and tricyclic antidepressants.

Respiratory Medicine

Multiple True/False Answers

199 E

Sweat tests require that the average collection of sweat should be over 1 g/m² per minute and that the sweat should only be collected for between 20 and 30 minutes.

The chloride concentration of the sweat must be measured – a result above 60 mmol/l is very suggestive of cystic fibrosis.

The Royal College of Paediatrics and Child Health has produced an appraisal of evidence-based guidelines for the performance of sweat tests for the investigation of cystic fibrosis in the UK; visit www.rcpch.ac.uk.

200 ABCDE

Other causes are:

- congenital central hypoventilation syndrome
- obesity
- inborn errors of metabolism
- neurodegenerative disorders.

201 ADE

Pulmonary presentations include pneumonia, repeated bronchiolitis, haemoptysis and chronic sinusitis.

Gastrointestinal presentations are:

- meconium ileus
- ileal atresia
- steatorrhoea
- rectal prolapse
- neonatal hepatitis
- hypoproteinaemia.

Miscellaneous presenting features include short stature and failure to thrive, diabetes mellitus, pseudo-Bartter syndrome and male infertility.

answers

202 D

Epiglottis is caused by *Haemophilus influenzae*, which has become uncommon since the introduction of the vaccination programme within the UK. Classically, the onset is sudden over a few hours, with the child being unable to swallow his or her own saliva because of the pain and hence sitting forward with the mouth open and drooling. The child appears toxic and often has a temperature of over 38–40°C, possibly also with a muffled stridor. IN NO CIRCUMSTANCES SHOULD THE CHILD BE UPSET AS COMPLETE OBSTRUCTION OF THE UPPER AIRWAY CAN OCCUR. Therefore, there should be no radiographs, no blood tests and no insertion of a cannula. Expert help should be sought and a calm environment maintained.

Best of Five Answer

203 A – A woman with human immunodeficiency virus (HIV) infection taking amphetamines

The risk factors for pulmonary arterial hypertension are:

- *Drugs*
  - Definite: aminorex, fenfluramine, dexfenfluramine, toxic rapeseed oil
  - Very likely: amphetamines, L-tryptophan
  - Possible: met-amphetamines, cocaine, chemotherapeutic agents
  - Unlikely: antidepressants, oral contraceptives, oestrogen therapy, cigarette smoking.
- *Demographic and medical conditions*
  - Definite: being female
  - Possible: pregnancy, systemic hypertension, splenectomy
  - Unlikely: obesity.
- *Diseases*
  - Definite: HIV
  - Very likely: portal hypertension, collagen vascular diseases, congenital systemic– pulmonary shunts (Eisenmenger's syndrome)
  - Possible: thyroid disorders, haemoglobinopathies, type 1a glycogen storage disease (von Gierke's disease), lipid storage disease (Gaucher's disease), hereditary haemorrhagic telangiectasia.

Reference: Seminar on primary pulmonary hypertension. *Lancet* 2003; **361**: 1533–1544.

204

1 **D – Sleep study**

2 **E – Obstructive sleep apnoea**

Risk factors for chronic obstructive sleep apnoea include craniofacial abnormalities, neurological sequelae including hydrocephalus, hypotonia and developmental delay, polycythaemia with sickle cell disease, obesity, large tonsils, myxoedema, cardiac failure, kyphoscoliosis and chronic asthma. Syndromes involved include Down's syndrome, Pickwickian syndrome, Ondine's curse and syndromes associated with obesity, including Prader–Willi syndrome. Other exacerbating factors include obstructed pharynx, acromegaly, small jaw, glycogen storage diseases, superior vena cava obstruction, enlarged adenoids and drug overdoses, including benzodiazepines, alcohol, sedatives and analgesics.

Investigations include a sleep study, audiovisual monitoring and polysonography; an ECG might show right ventricular hypertrophy. A sleep study will, however, provide the definitive diagnosis. Complications of undiagnosed chronic obstructive sleep apnoea include pulmonary and systemic hypertension, chronic cyanosis, cor pulmonale, right ventricular hypertrophy, polycythaemia and an increased incidence of road traffic accidents.

205

1 **A – Community-acquired pneumonia**

2 **D – *Streptococcus pneumoniae***

3 **E – Penicillin**

Pneumonia is very common in childhood, and on average every preschool child suffers from eight colds per year. Pneumonia is thought of in two categories: First, hospital-acquired *Streptococcus pneumoniae*, Gram-negative pneumonia, staphylococcal pneumonia, fungal pneumonia, *Haemophilus influenza* and *Legionella*. The most common bacterial agents are the group A β-haemolytic *Streptococcus* in adults and the group B β-haemolytic *Streptococcus* in neonates. *Klebsiella* is the most common cause of a Gram-negative pneumonia, producing cavitating lesions and pneumatocoeles. *Staphylococcus aureus* may cause cavitating lesions and is common where there is underlying lung pathology and congenital defects. Fungal pneumonia is often found in candidates at risk of malnutrition, failure to thrive, immunosuppression and chronic granulomatous disease. *Haemophilus* pneumonia is common in children less than 2 years of age and in those with pre-existing bronchitis.

answers

Recurrent chest infections may be due to IgG II and IgG IV deficiency. These children present with infections due to encapsulated polysaccharide organisms including *Haemophilus* and *Pneumococcus*. IgG I and IgG III act against protein antigens, whereas IgG II and IgG IV react against carbohydrate.

Second, community-acquired pneumonia is more common in the elderly and in children who are immunocompromised or suffer from heart failure. Possible causative organisms include *Streptococcus pneumoniae*, *Klebsiella*, *Coxiella* B, *Pneumococcus*, *Chlamydia psittaci*, *Mycoplasma*, *Mycobacterium tuberculosis*, adenovirus, measles, influenza, chicken pox and varicella zoster viruses but not *Bordetella* infections.

206

1   **C – Spiral computed tomography (CT) scan**

2   **C – Pulmonary embolism**

For various reasons, pulmonary embolism is becoming more common in paediatric practice. Factors include oral contraceptive pill and intravenous drug abuse, antithrombin III deficiency, protein S and C deficiency, hereditary thrombophilia and cardiac failure; more common causes include the use of central catheters, smoking, post-surgical immobilisation and bed rest, obesity, postpartum complications and a pelvic mass.

Investigations that may aid the diagnosis include a spiral CT scan. However, if this is not available, a radioisotope ventilation–perfusion scan will show mismatched ventilation and perfusion, although there is a high false-positive outcome. A normal ventilation–perfusion scan can rule out a pulmonary embolism but cannot confirm one. Angiography, combined with ventilation–perfusion isotope scans, a chest radiograph, an ECG and arterial blood gases will complete the investigations.

Extended Matching Answers

207 Theme: Pleural effusion

1   **F – Nephritic syndrome, G – Constrictive pericarditis, H – Peritoneal dialysis fluid**

2   **H – Peritoneal dialysis fluid**

3   **F – Nephritic syndrome**

Pleural effusions are thought of in four categories: (1) exudates, (2) transudates, (3) haemorrhagic and (4) straw-coloured.

Exudative pleural effusions are found when the protein concentration is >30 g/l with an LDH >200 iu/l. Causes include infections (tuberculosis), malignancies (Hodgkin's disease) and autoimmune diseases such as sarcoidosis, acute pancreatitis, pancreatic pseudocysts and asbestos exposure. Other rare causes include oesophageal perforation, Dressler's syndrome and yellow nail syndrome.

Transdusative pleural effusions are found when the protein concentration is <30 g/l with an LDH <200 iu/l. Causes include nephrotic syndrome, pseudomyxoedema, nephritic syndrome, peritoneal dialysis fluid, alcoholic cirrhosis of the liver, hypothyroidism, hyperproteinaemia, cystic fibrosis and constrictive pericarditis.

Causes of _haemorrhagic pleural effusions_ include haemothorax, trauma, secondary pancreatic disease, malignancy, pulmonary embolism and coagulopathy.

Causes of a _straw-coloured pleural effusion_ include nephritic syndrome and malignancies.

Coal-workers' pneumoconiosis is not associated with a pleural effusion. The glucose content of a pleural effusion is often low in rheumatoid disease, infection and malignancies, and the amylase level may be high in pancreatitis. Malignant cells may be present in only 50% of cases of malignancy, and blood-stained pleural effusion is not pathognomonic of malignancy. A chest radiograph does not exclude a pleural effusion as 200–300 ml is needed for an effusion to be detected. An ultrasound scan is beneficial, but ultimately a computed tomography scan will detect all levels of effusion.

208 Theme: Transfer factor

1   **A – Fever and increased metabolism**
     B – Anaemia
     D – Polycythaemia
     G – Increased pulmonary and capillary blood flow
     I – Pulmonary haemorrhage
     J – Athletes and increased exercise

2   **B – Anaemia**
     C – Pulmonary embolism
     E – Empyema
     F – Pulmonary hypertension
     H – Pneumonectomy

answers

3   **B – Anaemia**

Transfer factor can be raised by increases in haemodynamic circulation, haemoglobin level, pulmonary and capillary blood flow, carbon monoxide level, surface area of the lung and metabolic rate. Factors that lower the transfer factor include conditions that affect the lung parenchyma, decreased lung capillaries, ventilation–perfusion mismatch and shunts, and anaemia, and this may be improved by lobectomy, medical management of the disease and decreased blood flow to the lung.

Rheumatology

Multiple True/False Answers

209 AD

There must be a fever of at least 5 days' duration, with four out of the five following features (NB: only three of these are required if the patient has coronary artery aneurysm formation):

- diffuse, non-specific rash
- erythema of the hands and feet (which desquamates by days 14–21)
- cervical lymphadenopathy – often a solitary enlarged node of more than 1.5 cm in diameter
- involvement of the oral mucosa
- non-exudative conjunctivitis – under slit-lamp examination, there may be an anterior uveitis.

210 ABD

Discitis is seen most commonly in preschool children, who may present by refusing to flex the lumbar spine; other presentations include refusing to walk and limping. Back pain is also a common compliant. The condition is thought to be caused by an infection, especially with *Staphylococcus aureus*, and hence responds rapidly to antibiotic treatment. A radiograph can show a narrowed disc space and a variable amount of end-plate damage. Magnetic resonance imaging is the optimal imaging modality and will reveal the extent of involvement. Pain relief with antibiotic treatment is mandatory and must be continued for at least 6 weeks.

211 ACDE

Articular immune deposition is seen following meningococcal disease. Reiter's syndrome with plantar fasciitis is seen not only following sexually transmitted disease, but also after dysentery. Reactive arthropathy can also occur after streptococcal and viral infection. Infective causes of a monoarthropathy include: bacterial, viral, tubercular or fungal sources, or it may be caused by spirochaetes. Direct spread from adjacent osteomyelitis is well known to occur.

answers

Malignancy such as acute leukaemia, neuroblastoma or local bone/ cartilagenous tumours can cause a monoarthritis. Haematological abnormalities such as sickle cell disease and all forms of haemophilia are included in the list of causes, as is trauma, both accidental and non-accidental.

212 None is true

Perthes' disease occurs predominantly in children aged 4–9 years, boys being five times more likely to have this condition than girls. In this, there is avascular necrosis of the head of the femur, the condition being bilateral in only 15–18% of cases. The aetiology is unknown. Radiographs may initially appear normal; radionuclide bone scanning reveals a decreased uptake (this being increased in irritable hip), and magnetic resonance imaging best reveals early epiphyseal necrosis.

The course to resolution and healing can take several years, with preschool children having the best outcome. Femoral osteotomy is rarely required, but older children may need manipulation under general anaesthesia to ensure that the epiphysis remains within the acetabulum.

Best of Five Answers

213 B

Ankylosing spondylitis has an incidence of 1 in 2000 and presents usually under the age of 40 years. It is predominantly a disease of the adolescent years but may present under the age of 8. It is more prominent in boys, girls usually suffering a milder course of disease. There is often a 500-fold increase in the level of HLAB27. Not all patients show a positivity in this HLA antigen, and therefore it is not a diagnostic test.

Clinical characteristics include oligoarthritis, sacroileitis, aortitis, aortic regurgitation, anterior uveitis, conjunctivitis and acute iridocyclitis. Musculoskeletal abnormalities include calcified spinal ligaments, lumbosacral and iliac back pain, enthesopathy and a late presentation of bamboo spine. These children do not show any rheumatoid nodules, scleroderma or Gottron's papules. Complications include amyloidosis, nephrotic syndrome, atlanto-axial subluxation, syndesmophytes, enthesopathy, bamboo spine, Reiter's disease, aortic incompetence with conduction defects, acute pulmonary fibrosis, bronchiectasis and mild prostatitis. These children rarely present with a fever, osteoarthritis or myositis. Treatment options include non-steroidal anti-inflammatory drugs, sulfasalazine, physiotherapy, radiotherapy and ultimately joint replacement.

214 C

There is an increased incidence of Behçet's disease in Japan and the Middle East; it is thought that the disease ran along the old Silk Road from China to Turkey. There is an association with HLA B5, and 30% of cases have a positive family history. There is a male predominance of 20:1, and the disease is more common in the older age group of 20- to 40-year-olds, although it may present in adolescence. The clinical features include the triad of oral ulceration, genital ulceration and iritis. Other features include arthritis, arthropathy and uveitis. Around 10% may present with neurological sequelae and 25% with vascular thrombosis or a vasculitic thrombophlebitis; 50% of children may suffer from gastrointestinal complications. Dermatological features include pustules and papules, and 65% may present with erythema nodosum. There is no evidence of alopecia, keratoderma or blenorrhoea. HLA B27 is associated with ankylosing spondylitis, HLA DRW2 with systemic lupus erythematosus, HLA B35 with subacute thyroiditis and HLA QW2 with coeliac disease.

215 E

DIL is common in boys, unlike idiopathic SLE, for which there is a predominance in girls of 9:1. DIL may show positivity to single-stranded DNA and affects slow acetylators. Patients may show a positive ANA serology result. Antihistone antibody may be positive, and anti-Ro antibody may cause nephritis. Single-stranded DNA may cause an associated SLE, and anti-Ro and anti-La antibodies may exacerbate neonatal lupus. Drugs that may induce a lupus-type reaction include sulphonamides, isoniazid, griseofulvin, hydralazine, propylthiouracil, penicillamine, procainamide and carbamazepine. Clinically, DIL reactions are those of an allergic reaction with an SLE component, namely facial rash, erythema and arthralgia. They are virtually never complicated by renal or neurological disease, and withdrawal of the drug leads to disappearance of the disease. Complete reversal may take up to 2 years.

216 E

The autosomal dominant disorder of achondroplasia has a risk of recurrence of future generations of 50%. The homozygous autosomal recessive type is lethal. The abnormality is caused by a mutation of the FGFR3 gene on chromosome 4. Mutations of chromosome 4 have been identified in hypochondroplasia and other skeletal dysplasias; the effects are thought to arise from a mutation within the FGFR1 and FGFR2 genes. The pathophysiology may be that of defective endochondrial bone formation with normal membranous bone development. The vault of the

answers

skull, which is membranous, grows at the normal rate, but the limb bones, which are endochondrial, are stunted.

Other clinical phenotypes include normal healthy bones, a normal skull circumference, a disproportionately short stature with broad and short limbs, lumbar lordosis, thoracic kyphosis and short hands and fingers. The abnormal facial development causes an increased incidence of otitis media, conductive hearing loss and chronic obstructive sleep apnoea. These children have normal skin, a normal IQ and normal sexual characteristics. Other complications include early osteoarthritis, hydrocephalus, paraplegia, foramen magnum compression and obstetric difficulties. The differential diagnosis includes achondrogenesis and atrophic dysplasia, Ellis–van Creveld's syndrome and hyperchondroplasia.

217 C

SLE is a multisystem disease that causes widespread inflammation of the connective tissues and an immune complex vasculitis. It commonly presents in childhood with lupus nephritis in girls (3:1 ratio of girls:boys). It is uncommon under the age of 5 years, and only 20% present in childhood. SLE has an increased incidence in adolescent girls (10:1) and is less common in Caucasians but prominent in dark-skinned people.

The World Health Organisation (WHO) has classified SLE into five classes, and the clinical presentation may be either insidious or acute. Other clinical features noted include symmetrical arthritis, non-erosive arthropathy, arthralgia, myalgia, myositis, serositis and Raynaud's phenomenon. Joint deformities are uncommon. Glomerulonephritis is found in 50% of patients. Both nephrotic and nephritic syndrome may progress to chronic renal failure. Alopecia, a photosensitivity rash, dermatitis, livido reticularis and benign subacute cutaneous disease may be noted. Children may present acutely with pleurisy or pleural effusion, and on investigation small pulmonary nodules with pulmonary fibrosis may be seen. Peritonitis, intussusception, pericarditis, myocarditis, hypertension and fatal myocardial infarction are associated. Antiphospholipid antibody-positive patients may present with unilateral blindness. These patients must be supervised as they are prone to psychotic and depressive states.

Investigations may show marrow aplasia, and radiology confirms the absence of erosions, avascular necrosis being more common in children than adults.

218

1   **A – ANA (ANA) antibody positive**

2   **E – All of the above**

3   **C – Neonatal lupus**

Neonatal lupus presents in the neonatal period and is acquired transplacentally. It is associated with maternal anti-Ro and anti-La antibodies. These antibodies are also found in maternal SLE and Sjögren's syndrome, but there is no associated clinical disease. Neonatal lupus may present as a syndrome with a triad of dermatitis, thrombocytopenia and congenital heart block. Clinical presentation may vary, and other clinical features include dermatitis, thrombocytopenia, autoimmune haemolytic anaemia, hepatic fibrosis, hepatitis, hepatosplenomegaly and pulmonary fibrosis.

Investigations include a cardiac echo (to exclude congenital heart disease), A and E antibody serology (positive), rheumatoid factor (negative) and anti-double-stranded DNA antibody (negative). A maternal blood sample may show positivity to Ro and La antibodies and double-stranded DNA antibody. The only antenatal treatment option is dexamethasone. The prognosis suggests that there is resolution before 9 months of age.

Extended Matching Answer

219 Theme: Vasculitides

1   **C – ANCA positive**

Polyarteritis nodosa is predominantly a renal disease that involves all three layers of the arterial wall. Renal failure is secondary to hypertension, thrombosis, infarction, aneurysms, and necrotising arteritis. Necrotising proliferative glomerulonephritis with crescentic formation is often found. Other complications include aneurysms, organ infarction and neuropathy. ANCA positivity is found in 50% of cases.

2   **A – Perinuclear antinuclear cytoplasmic antibody (ANCA) positive**

Microscopic polyangiitis is more common in males. It involves microscopic disease and complications involve pulmonary and renal disease. Peripheral ANCA positivity is found in 50–60% of patients.

answers

3   **E – Cytoplasmic ANCA positive**

Wegener's granulomatosis is more common in males. It affects the arterioles and veins, and complications include vascular granulomata, necrotising vasculitis, respiratory disease, renal disease, otitis media, proptosis and mononeuritis multiplex. Cytoplasmic ANCA positivity is found in 80% of cases.

Statistics

Multiple True/False Answers

220 E

The NNT is the number of patients out of all those treated who obtain benefit from that treatment. It is the inverse of the absolute risk reduction, which relates to the difference in risk of something happening between the patients in the control group and those in the treatment group.

The relative risk is the proportion of the original risk still present in the treatment group and is worked out as the treatment risk of an event divided by the control group risk of the same event occurring.

The odds ratio is the proportion of patients with a target event divided by the proportion without a target event.

The number-needed-to-harm is the number of patients who suffer from the treatment out of all the patients who are treated.

221 ABCD

Selection bias refers to how the subject was chosen to be studied; the omission of patients may have a significant effect on the study. Similarly, bias will arise if patients are not randomly allocated to groups.

Proportionately fewer studies with negative results are published, which may alter the perception of the true effects of a treatment when considering the literature as a whole.

Increased patient motivation in those who have suffered an event may also influence the results, as may the researchers themselves, by searching harder in the group who have experienced an event than in the control group.

Blinding is an important technique to remove treatment bias – double-blinding being when neither the patients nor the staff looking after them are aware of the treatment regimes that the patients are receiving.

answers

The patients who are lost to follow-up have been found in many studies (ones that have gone to seek them out) to include a disproportionately large number of patients who have had an event compared with the rest of that group who were not lost to follow-up.

222 None is true

Confidence intervals tend to be smaller the larger the sample size and give an idea of the range of the mean that has been found from the study. The 5% and 95% values are commonly used, but any interval can be chosen. The confidence interval tends to be given about a mean.

223 A

Probability of the diagnosis

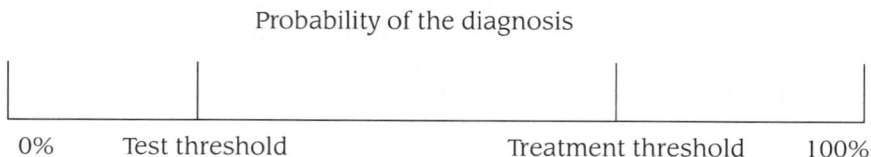

0%   Test threshold   Treatment threshold   100%

Figure 6 Diagnostic test thresholds

The probability at which a clinician decides that investigation is not warranted is the test threshold; this is a variable figure (Figure 6). The treatment threshold is the value at which a test is not warranted as the diagnosis is clinically very likely; again there is no fixed probability ascribed to this figure. The patient's condition alters the likelihood of whether a test should be carried out.

224 C

The probability is the measure of the likely proportion of events having a particular outcome in a large series of experiments. For example, a disease state for which there is no known sex difference, the probability that the next patient presenting with the disease is 50%, 0.5 or 1/20.

Probability values lie between 0 and 1 inclusive.

- If $p = 0$ then the outcome never occurs
- If $p = 1$ then the outcome will always occur without fail
- If $p = 0.5$ then the outcome will occur in 50% of experiments
- 0.01 is less significant compared to 0.001
- 1% is less significant compared to 0.01%
- 1/100 is less significant compared to 1/1000.

Prior probability:
This is the theoretical chance of having the disease if the patient is simply in the population, ie the probability of getting the disease.

Posterior probability:
This is the empirical chance of having the disease following a test for that disease. It depends on how good the test is. If the test is excellent it changes the posterior probability a lot.

225 E

Standard deviation is the square root of the variance squared.

Standard error of the mean reflects the sampling error in calculating the population mean. It is a measure of the likely accuracy of the sample mean. It measures the scatter of data around the mean. The standard error of the mean must be smaller than the SD. The sample error and the standard error are often used to compute the confidence interval, which has a stated probability of including the true population mean. SE is NOT used to calculate the chi-squared test as it compares proportions and is NOT related to the SD. The SD and SE may only be used in a normally distributed population.

$$SE = \frac{SD}{N}.$$

Best of Five Answer

226 A

Correlation methods are used to determine the strength of the linear mathematical relationship between two continuous variables measured on a single group of individuals. The correlation coefficient describes how well data fit the proposed regression line. It should not be computed if the relationship is not thought to be linear.

The parametric Pearson correlation coefficient, R, is used if one or both variables have a normal distribution. R is used to determine if there is a mathematical linear relationship between diastolic blood pressure and serum cholesterol levels in a group of patients with hypertension.

The non-parametric Spearman or Kendall rank correlation coefficient is used if neither variable has a normal distribution or the sample size is small (ie <20).

answers

Facts are:

- The correlation coefficient takes values between −1 and 1 inclusive.
- It depicts an increase in one variable accompanied by a related increase in another.
- A significant correlation does not imply a cause and effect.

Extended Matching Answers

227 Theme: Diagnostic tests

1 **A – Specificity**

2 **C – Positive predictive value**

3 **G – Incidence**

Diagnostic tests are best discussed as definitions and the following diagram:

Diagnostic test result	Diseased	Disease-free
Positive (indicating possible disease)	a	b
Negative	c	d

a. Sensitivity

This is the proportion of TRUE POSITIVES that are correctly identified by a test and have true negatives and a few false-negatives. It tells us about FALSE NEGATIVES. This category is good at picking up a disease.

$$\frac{a}{a+c}$$

b. Specificity

This is the proportion of TRUE NEGATIVES that are correctly identified by a test and have true positives and a few false-positives. It tells us about the FALSE POSITIVES. This category is good at excluding a disease.

$$\frac{d}{b+d}$$

c. Positive predictive value

This category determines those that have a positive test and determines how many truly have the disease, ie true-positives and test-positive results. This depicts the chance that you may have the condition if your test result is positive.

$$\frac{a}{a+b}$$

d. Negative predictive value

This category determines those that have a negative test and determines how many truly do not have the disease, ie true-negatives and test-negative results. This depicts the chance that you may not have the condition if your test result is negative.

$$\frac{d}{c+d}$$

In general if a high number of patients with a positive result are correctly diagnosed as having the disease then the test has a high positive predictive value. A good test has a high sensitivity and a high negative predictive value. A specific and sensitive test is good for screening.

e. Precision

The precision of an assay is one in which repeated observations conform to themselves.

f. Accuracy

The accuracy of observations is the closeness of the observations to the quality intended to be measured.

g. Incidence

The incidence is the number of new cases diagnosed per head of population in a given time, usually one year. A longitudinal study is used to determine this figure.

h. Prevalence

The prevalence is the number of cases suffering from a disease per head of population in a time given, usually one year. A cross-sectional study is used to determine this figure.

i. Attack rate

The attack rate for a given disease is the proportion of people exposed to infections that then go on to develop the disease.

answers

228 Theme: Clinical trials

1 **C – Double-blind placebo-controlled trial**

2 **G – Crossover trial**

3 **F – Parallel trial**

In a clinical trial it is easier to show that there is a difference between two treatments than no difference. The smaller the p number the less the numerical difference between groups means.

1 **Blind trial**
   a One or more parties are unaware of the treatment being administered.

2 **Single-blind trial**
   a The patient alone is unaware of the treatment being administered

3 **Double-blind trial**
   a The patient and the doctor are unaware of the treatment being administered.
   b Double-blind is better compared to single-blind studies.

4 **Triple-blind trial**
   a The patient, the doctor and a third party are unaware of the treatment being administered.

5 **Double-blind placebo-controlled trial**
   a The patient and the doctor are unaware as to who receives the drug in question and who receives a placebo. A placebo is a pharmacologically inactive substance given as if it were the active agent. Most patients will exhibit the placebo response and appear to respond to treatment with the inactive agent. Colours to avoid for placebo medication are blue and green as these are perceived as poisons. Capsules with a red, brown or yellow colour give a better response.
   b The placebo effect is very important.

6 **Parallel trial**
   a This clinical trial is conducted in a parallel fashion so that each patient is exposed to a single treatment only.
   b Multi-centre designs are recommended to obtain sufficient cases.

7 **Cross-over trial**
   a This clinical trial occurs when each patient is exposed to both treatments therefore allowing comparisons of each treatment. Fewer patients are needed compared to that of a parallel trial.
   b These trials are best used for drugs with a short-term duration of onset of action, other words a short-term in relief of chronic symptoms.
   c In these studies a period of 'wash-out' is essential to eradicate potential carry-over effects before commencing the second treatment.

8 Controlled trial

a The role of ethics is there to protect the patient

b Patient bias is more likely if the response is subjective

c A random double-blind test may be unnecessary

d For most studies the random sample size is not present

e Where a treatment can cure previous fatal illnesses a controlled trial is not required

f Stratification tries to match groups for a number of equal factors, eg sex, smoking status.

9 Randomisation

a This ensures that the allocated treatment for each patient is a matter of chance. Randomisation may be dealt with by computer allocation, flipping a coin, and the proposed trail agent delivered via a sealed closed envelope.

Vaccination

Multiple True/False Answers

229 ABC

Other definite contraindications include a severe adverse reaction to a previous immunisation, general reactions including fever of over 39.5°C, anaphylaxis, laryngeal spasm and a severe local reaction with greater than 50% circumferential erythema and swelling of the injected limb.

230 BC

Patients receiving treatment for TB can be given live vaccines. Live vaccines are inactivated by a normal dose of immunoglobulin, hence they cannot be given within 3 months after immunoglobulins are given as the effects may be modified. Organ-transplanted patients may be receiving immunosuppressive regimes; similarly, human immunodeficiency virus-infected or steroid-receiving patients should not be given live vaccines. Prematurity or jaundice in the neonatal period is not a contraindication.

231 E

The Hib vaccine was introduced into the UK in 1992. It is a conjugate vaccine that has been very successful in decreasing the incidence of invasive *Haemophilus influenzae* type B infections. The vaccine has decreased the incidence of epiglottitis, meningitis and otitis media in our population.

232 B

Children with sickle cell disease are at increased risk of *Haemophilus* and *Pneumococcus* infections and therefore must be protected with the Hib vaccine as part of their treatment protocol. The vaccine has no effect on staphylococcal infections, septic arthritis or periorbital cellulitis. Children with asplenia and those who have recently had a splenectomy are offered the pneumovax vaccine.

Extended Matching Answers

233 Theme: Vaccination schedule

1 **I – BCG**
2 **A – DTP 3, B – Polio 3, C – Meningitis C 3, D – Hib 3**
3 **F – BCG**

The current immunisation protocols for children are shown in Table 15.

DPT/polio	2, 3, 4 months
Hib/meningitis C	2, 3, 4 months
DPT/meningitis C/polio booster	4–5 years preschool
DPT/meningitis C/polio booster	15–18 years leaving school
Hib	13–14 months single dose if not previously given. It is not recommended if the child is >4 years of age
MMR	12–18 months
MMR booster	3–5 years
Rubella booster	10–14 years in girls who have not had previous MMR vaccination
BCG	At birth if from a tuberculosis-endemic area
	10–14 years

Table 15: Current immunisation protocols

234 Theme: Contraindications to vaccination

1 **A – Encephalitis**
   D – Previous seizures
   H – Shock

DPT is contraindicated if a child has had previous seizures or if there is a previous history of anaphylaxis, collapse or shock. Pertussis infection is not a contraindication and is a COMPLICATION of the DPT vaccine.

2 **B – High-dose corticosteroids**
   C – An infant of, or a mother with, human immunodeficiency virus (HIV)
   E – A positive tuberculin test
   F – Immunocompromised host
   I – Disseminated BCGosis

answers

Contraindications for giving live vaccines are:

- high-dose corticosteroid treatment
- immunosuppressive treatment
- receiving the vaccination within 3 months of receiving intravenous immunoglobulin
- untreated malignancy
- immune-deficient states, ie hypogammaglobulinaemia
- involvement with the sibling or parent of a child in an immunocompromised state
- HIV-positive patient
- infant of a mother with HIV
- pregnancy
- an acute febrile illness at the time of immunisation
- a positive tuberculin skin test
- a general septic skin condition
- disseminated BCG
- if the child has received another live vaccine within 3 weeks prior to this
- anaphylaxis in response to a previous vaccine
- egg anaphylaxis.

3   **C – An infant of, or a mother with, human immunodeficiency virus (HIV)**
     F – Immunocompromised host

The side-effects of BCG vaccination include swelling and erythema, skin ulceration and abscess at the site. BCGosis and regional adenitis are often found in patients with atopy, eczema and an immunocompromised state. Contraindications for giving the BCG vaccination include an infant or a mother with HIV, and if the child has an immunocompromised state or is currently taking steroids. The live BCG and conjugated Hib vaccines may be given together. BCG vaccine can be given with any concurrent live vaccine but NOT at the same time, ie there must be a 3-week interval between vaccines, and each vaccine must be given into a different arm. A 3-month interval is required if the same arm is used.

235 Theme: Live and attenuated vaccines

1   **C – Yellow fever**
     D – MMR
     F – Polio (Sabin)
     H – Live attenuated typhoid

The following are live vaccines: MMR, single measles, single mumps, single rubella, polio (Sabin), yellow fever, varicella zoster virus (ZIG), BCG and live attenuated typhoid.

2   **A – Polio (Salk)**
     B – Cholera
     E – Pneumococcal
     G – Polysaccharide typhoid
     I – Hib
     J – Hepatitis B

The following are killed inactivated vaccines: *Bordetella pertussis*, diphtheria, tetanus, polio (Salk), polysaccharide typhoid, cholera, hepatitis B, Hib and pneumococcal.

3   **F – Polio (Sabin), H – Live attenuated typhoid**

236 Theme: Identifying vaccines

1   **D – Measles**
     F – Rubella

The MMR vaccine is given irrespective of whether the child has previously had measles, mumps or rubella. It is not given in the first trimester of pregnancy as it is associated with a high incidence of abortion. The single measles, mumps or rubella vaccine is a live vaccine that has recently been used when parents have refused to allow the MMR combined vaccine. It is given at 12–18 months of age, irrespective of any previous history of illness, and at 10–14 years of age as a booster to all girls. The vaccine can be given within 72 hours of exposure to measles and can prevent the disease occurring. The vaccine has, however, a higher morbidity rate than the DPT vaccine. The side-effects of the measles vaccine are the same as for any other live vaccine.

2   **H – Polio (Sabin)**

The live (Sabin) polio vaccine is an attenuated virus strain and is the most common cause of polio-related paralysis in the UK. The oral version is NOT superior to the intramuscular version. The oral vaccine does NOT cause transient diarrhoea but it does cause excretion of polio organisms in the stool and therefore must not be given to the siblings of children who are immunocompromised. This vaccine must be given to children who are breastfeeding, have an immune deficiency or are born to a mother infected with human immunodeficiency virus. The inactivated (Salk) polio vaccine is given intramuscularly and is now routinely given with the vaccines at 2, 3 and 4 months respectively.

3   **A – Varicella zoster immunoglobulin (ZIG)**

The varicella zoster immunoglobulin (ZIG) must be given to all children who are immunocompromised and have been in contact with a child with chicken pox or shingles. The siblings of children who are immunocompromised must also be vaccinated. The vaccine is

answers

contraindicated in the first trimester of pregnancy, must not be given at the same time as other live vaccines and must be withheld if the child has varicella zoster syndrome.

Index

Locators are given as question number.

PASTEST – DEDICATED TO YOUR SUCCESS

PasTest has been publishing books for medical students and doctors for over 30 years. Our extensive experience means that we are always one step ahead when it comes to knowledge of current trends in undergraduate exams.

We use only the best authors, which enables us to tailor our books to meet your revision needs. We incorporate feedback from candidates to ensure that our books are continually improved.

This commitment to quality ensures that students who buy PasTest books achieve successful exam results.

Delivery to your door
With a busy lifestyle, nobody enjoys walking to the shops for something that may or may not be in stock. Let us take the hassle and deliver direct to your door. We will dispatch your book within 24 hours of receiving your order.

How to Order:
www.pastest.co.uk
To order books safely and securely online, shop at our website.

Telephone: +44 (0)1565 752000 Fax: +44 (0)1565 650264
For priority mail order.
Have your credit card to hand when you call.

Write to us at:
PasTest Ltd
Egerton Court
Parkgate Industrial Estate
Knutsford
WA16 8DX

PASTEST BOOKS FOR PAEDIATRICS

PasTest are the specialists in study guides and revision courses for medical qualifications. For over 30 years we have been helping doctors to achieve their potential. The PasTest range of books for postgraduate paediatric exams includes:

Essential Revision Notes in Paediatrics for the MRCPCH
Mark Beattie and Mike Champion
ISBN: 1 901198 64 2

Basic Child Health Practice Papers
First Para:Peter De Halpert and Ian Pollock
ISBN: 1 904627 08 0

Essential Questions in Paediatrics for MRCPCH 1 Volumes 1&2
Mark Beattie and Mike Champion
ISBN: Volume 1 – 1 901198 99 5
         Volume 2 – 1 904627 33 1

MRCPCH Part 1 Paediatric MCQs with Individual Subject Summaries 2nd edition
Mark Beattie
ISBN: 1 901198 50 2

Questions for the MRCPCH Part 2 Written Examination
Nick Barnes and Julian Forton
ISBN: 1 904627 16 1

MRCPCH Part 2 Practice Exams 3rd edition
Giles Kendall and Ian Pollock
ISBN: 1 901198 87 1

Short Cases for the Paediatric Membership
Mark Beattie, Andrew Clark and Anne Smith
ISBN: 1 901198 25 1

For further information about these titles, visit our website at www.pastest.co.uk